Thumbs Up

How to Survive Without Your Smartphone for

24 Hours

Michael Macleod and Matthew Milne

ISBN-13: 978-1508827412
ISBN-10: 1508827419

24hourThumbsUp@gmail.com
www.24hourThumbsUp.com

For those of us who love our smartphones

a bit too much.

"We're so busy watching out for what's just ahead of us that we don't take time to enjoy where we are."

Bill Watterson, creator of Calvin and Hobbes

"We need to be smarter than our smart phones and realize the people we are with are more important than the people we aren't with, and way more important than the strangers we hope will tweet and like and share."

Regina Brett

"Technology... the knack of so arranging the world that we don't have to experience it."

Max Frisch

"Getting information off the Internet is like taking a drink from a fire hydrant."

Mitchell Kapor

Contents

Introduction - Switching off!

The realization - a case of the niggles.

If you're like me (or, you know, everyone else) then right now your phone is within easy reach — on your desk, in your pocket, or lying right beside you.

Sometimes I wonder just what on earth I did before I had a smartphone. How did I *survive*? How did I find my way around, stay in touch and keep myself entertained!?

I mean, you can rely on this palm-sized marvel of technology to do almost anything. And we do. We've found a way to use our phones in every situation. It's totally normal to dive in for five minutes here, ten minutes there, a game, a quick news article, email, send-reply-send-reply, music on the subway, WhatsApp,

Facebook, check Twitter feed...

But I often wonder if this constant attachment to my phone isn't limiting me in ways I'm not even aware of – maybe it's hijacked my brain...all these little distractions, these tugs at my attention - they all add up. I often get this scattered feeling, like I'm a little bit everywhere, but never fully somewhere.

Of course, I push this niggle to the back of my mind, telling myself: "Everyone's doing it. That's just how life is now." But it wouldn't go away. The niggle kept niggling.

And I wasn't the only one who felt this way. Many people I shared my thoughts with agreed – the niggles were for real!

The idea for this book first came about during a Skype conversation with Michael (co-author and illustrator of this book). We were joking about needing some sort of a 'smartphone detox.' Fired up by this idea we came up with a quick 'So you think you're not a smartphone addict' test. Here are some of the questions on it.

1. You are in the middle of a conversation and your phone starts buzzing, so you...
   - Ignore it and carry on talking.
   - Pause the conversation and check your phone.

- Pretend to pay attention while you check your phone.

2. When you go to the bathroom you take your phone with you, obviously, so you can tweet while you tinkle or post while you poop.
   - True. Love it!
   - False. Ewww!
   - Sometimes, sure.

3. You are pro at texting a friend while simultaneously conducting a real life conversation with your mom, or whoever.
   - True. My skills are legendary.
   - False. One thing at a time.
   - Well, I *do* text and chat sometimes.

4. You've experienced 'appnesia' or 'browser blackout.' You know, where you tell yourself: "Just one quick YouTube video before I start working." But after that first video you think "okay just one more..." And then somehow it's an hour later and you've just watched a hundred videos of cats climbing curtains.
   - True.
   - It wasn't cats, okay!

- Nope, that's never happened. I have the discipline of a battle-hardened samurai.

5. How many apps have you downloaded on your phone? How often do you use them? How much time do you spend searching for new apps, or better ones, or browsing what is available?
   - Just a few essentials.
   - All the latest stuff! There's always a better version.
   - I've downloaded far more apps than I actually use…

By the way, visit Smartphone Addiction Test Facility #746 at **https://24hourthumbsup.typeform.com/to/a2FDiy** to test your level of addiction!

The 'addiction test' was meant as a bit of lighthearted fun, but as we went over the examples we looked at each other. We were using our phones far more often than we realized - heck, maybe we *did* need a detox!

That was when Michael and I decided to make ourselves guinea pigs in our own experiment…

The experience - going Thumbs Up.

We dared each other to put aside our smartphones for 24 hours. And then we immediately ramped up the challenge. Because we wanted to make this more than a mere 'digital detox.' We wanted to address the feeling of disconnection our phones so often caused us – we wanted to cure the niggles!

So we challenged each other to be more productive, more connected and have more fun than on a regular day. We decided that every time we felt the urge to check our smartphones for notifications, every time we had some free time because we'd *normally* be playing a game or using an app or otherwise be a thumbs down, dead-to-the-world phone zombie – in these moments we would instead do something awesome. This is where we would take action and get engaged in something meaningful. Even if that just meant helping an old lady hobble across the street.

We dubbed our commitment the '24 hour Thumbs Up challenge' and established 2 rules:

1. Thumbs up and off your smartphone for a full 24 hours.

2. Every time you're tempted to use your smartphone, or at any time you'd normally be using it, you have to do something awesome instead - in the REAL world!

We agreed to 'go Thumbs Up' first thing the very next morning. We grinned at each other over Skype. CHALLENGE ACCEPTED!

Here are some of the highlights of my day. Keep in mind, I was teaching English in Korea at the time, so I relied *heavily* on my smartphone to translate things, get around and feel 'connected.'

I woke up and managed to turn my phone off without any difficulties. But during breakfast I kept glancing at the black screen. I'd usually scroll through news headlines while I ate. This was no good. I couldn't let Michael beat me so easily! Impulsively I yanked open my cupboard and shoved my phone under some pants. Ha - take that! I AM IN CONTROL! I sat down at the table again and focused my attention on eating my breakfast. My bacon and eggs have never tasted so yummy.

At work I usually spent a good portion of my lunch break playing Words with Friends on my phone. Today I didn't have that option. I decided to spend this time with my students instead. We started using this time for extra revision and it soon became a daily habit.

It was far more fun (and fulfilling) than tapping away at my phone. Besides, we ended up inventing our own word games!

That evening I met up with a friend for dinner. I explained my Thumbs Up challenge to her. She laughed and decided to play along, promising to not touch her phone for the rest of the night. Usually we'd scour blogs for a recommendation and then try to hunt the place down with Google Maps. Instead we began exploring the neighborhood for ourselves. Soon we were having an adventure, ducking down side alleys and being tempted by a whole range of new sights and smells. We stumbled across a cozy, family run restaurant without a hint of English on the menu. We resisted the reflex to rely on Google Translate. Instead we decided to be bold and order a bunch of unfamiliar items just to see what they were. And so we chanced across an unsung culinary wonderment: *gun mandu* - deep fried dumplings! Yesness!

After dinner I flagged down a taxi. During the ride home I found myself searching for my phone. This was my reflex behavior, another space I routinely filled with distraction. But now my phone was in my cupboard. Under some pants. So I decided to practice my fledgling Korean with the driver. He chuckled at my pronunciation and responded with his own broken English, grinning crazily at me in the rear-view mirror. When I told him I was from South Africa he immediately quipped: "Ah, Mandela! Good!"

He followed this with the hilarious: "Your country dangerous, bang bang! Korea very safe. Stay Korea!"

He proceeded to show me a series of photos of every member of his family ever, handing them back over the seat to me.

Pretty cool, eh?

These are some of Mike's highlights:

I always started my mornings with a twenty minute rundown of my social media feeds. Today, however, I couldn't – I was going Thumbs Up. I paced around my room for a minute, wondering what I might be missing out on. Then I thought: "So what? Those notifications aren't going anywhere. How can I use this time productively?"

I'd been meaning to start working out in the mornings for months now, but somehow I couldn't quite find the time for it. Well, that's what I told myself. Suddenly I realized I'd found the time!

Right then and there I dropped down and started doing push-ups. Afterwards I felt energized and alive. Why? It was so clear to me – I'd just done something I'd been putting off for ages!

At work I had another epiphany. Without my phone there were no interruptions during my tasks, nothing to take my attention off the project I was busy with.

I couldn't distract myself between tasks either. The temptation to quickly check email or scroll through Facebook was simply not there - I was able to stay focused and move right from one job to the next. I got through two days of work in a matter of hours. It was like Neo realizing he's The One. Usually checking my phone would result in three to ten minute 'breaks' every half hour. This was wasted time, and totally unnecessary. After each break it would take me another few minutes to get back into the swing of things. It was so simple: no phone = no breaks = I got stuff done fast!

Going Thumbs Up forced me to see where my phone was using me instead of me using it.

That evening I really wanted to share my phone-free experience with someone. Normally I'd just jump onto Facebook or Instagram. How could I do this without breaking the rules of my Thumbs Up challenge? Sure, I could've just used my computer, but that felt like cheating. We'd decided to make this day more meaningful than usual...

I started laughing as an idea struck me. I dug the telephone directory out of the storage closet and looked up an old buddy's landline number. He's as tech-obsessed as I am so I thought he'd be the perfect guy to share this story with.

He was surprised to hear from me on a 'telephone.' We joked about how old-school it was to be holding these huge receivers. Then we had an hour long debate about the evolution of mobile phones! Of course, if I had my smartphone I could have just called him, but here's the thing – I wouldn't have. I would have just sent a WhatsApp message. I realized I often forget about the 'phone' part of my smartphone.

The revelation – what you'll gain.

What we discovered was, well, exactly what we want you to discover. We know you're going to get a lot out of this book and we're super excited to hear about your experience. So please let us know how it went AFTER you've completed the challenge.

The 24 hour challenge will get you to see where your smartphone is improving your life and where it *isn't*. It will get you to see when you need your phone and when you really can do without it. You'll have those vital "A-ha!" moments where you realize how much time and energy you've been spending on turning yourself into a mindless phone zombie. And by finding these moments and replacing them with meaningful activities you're going to upgrade your life.

You'll discover, as we did, how great it is to be out there doing your own thing instead of looking at pictures and posts of other people living it up. Not having your phone on you will ensure you fully experience the moment, without distractions. And if you have some truly epic stories to share, as we're sure you will, you can always post about them after the challenge!

We found the greatest joys of the challenge came from *doing* things which made us be more productive, feel more connected and just have some good old fashioned fun. This is the heart and soul of the Thumbs Up challenge.

The rest of this book is dedicated to sparking those moments. It's designed as a treasure chest of activity ideas to get you adding highlights to your own challenge.

Because the point of going Thumbs Up is not just to survive for 24 hours, it's to *thrive*!

As you go over the activities in the following chapters, you might start thinking: "I could do this with my phone on!"

It's true - you could. But *would* you?

Going Thumbs Up is about creating opportunities which *wouldn't* happen if you had your phone handy…it's about embracing the unusual and forcing the unexpected. And this is the heart of the adventure — all those things which just wouldn't happen when you rely on apps and maps and taps on a tiny screen.

Because when you're permanently reliant on Yelp you miss out on all those truly special places, the ones you chance across as you explore the neighborhood with your friends.

Because when you're hunched over Google Maps you don't experience the journey from 'here' to 'that awesome cupcake café with the jiving jazz band.'

That said, we're not some smelly hippies who want you to get rid of your phone. That's ridiculous — smartphones are awesome and they do add immense value to our lives.

In today's world it's impossible to completely distance yourself from the digital. But the vision for the Thumbs Up challenge does run deeper than the first phone-free day. It's also about integrating the benefits and insights of your detox once you've picked up your smartphone again.

That's why we've started a blog at **www.24hourThumbsUp.com** to keep you up-to-date with new ideas for offline activities, share stories about digital detox lifestyles and to remind you to go Thumbs Up every now and then!

So this is it.

We'd like you to join us on an adventure.

Yes, it's going to force you to step out of your comfort zone.

Yes, it's going to be challenging (and awesome), but that's what you were expecting when you began it.

Because you have in fact already taken the first step. You wouldn't be reading this if you hadn't.

So let's take the second step.

The adventure you're about to have, the one you began when you opened this book, is going to re-acquaint you with the real. It's going to re-kindle a sense of connection with the world around you – and most importantly – the people around you. It's going to make you notice all the little things which get lost when your nose is pressed up against that smartphone screen.

And the method is simple. Action is the key. Turn the page and let's go Thumbs Up!

Here's how this is going to work...

Explanation – how the book is structured:

The chapters which follow consist of lists of activity prompts.

Treat them as little nuggets of inspiration. They're there to pop ideas into your head and get you to jump right in.

Because without the distractions offered by your smartphone, you'll have the time and attention to pour into actually *doing* some awesome things, both big and small.

Your Thumbs Up challenge is all about taking action, about *living* instead of being stuck behind a tiny screen. By taking action, by completing as many of the activities as possible you'll transform your detox into a series of practical life upgrades.

The activity lists in each chapter are grouped into three sections (not necessarily in the order they appear below).

- **Connection** activities will get you engaging and interacting with people. They're there to satisfy all those Facebook cravings.
- The **Productivity** section will channel your time into – wait for it – productive activities. Imagine if all those minutes you spend playing Candy Crush were poured into something constructive...you could totally be the master of *anything* by now! This section will get you started. 'Coz you've got to start somewhere.
- Lastly, **Entertainment**. Here you get to have oodles of fun. By actually doing stuff that requires more than two thumbs and glazed eyes!

These three sections are like three 'moods' – choose an activity based on your vibe at the time. You're welcome to jump around between sections!

The chapters themselves are each based on a time of day and

have been named accordingly. They'll guide you from the minute you wake up until the minute you go to bed.

Action – what you have to do:

You are going to have a truly kick-ass day. Guaranteed. But the onus is on YOU.

Your task is simple – use this book as a reference. Skim the relevant chapter and choose activities to complete. Try to do as many as possible!

There is no need to read through the entire book all at once – just stick to one chapter at a time, or simply be guided by your mood and focus on either the Connection, Entertainment or Productivity section inside of a chapter.

We've purposefully kept the chapters short. The activities descriptions are punchy and to-the-point. We don't want to keep you reading – we want you to be using this book as a springboard. Make the activities your own! The point is to *take* the initiative, to *start* on a project, to just *do do do!* Don't linger over the choice, just make one and then get right on it!

(An aside: if you're really struggling to complete the 24hourThumbsUp challenge, jump to the 'SOS' chapter at the very end of the book.)

Preparation – before you get started:

I recommend starting your Thumbs Up challenge from the beginning of a new day so these preparation tasks should be completed the night *before* you start.

- Post a cryptic status on Facebook and Twitter:
  "See you on the other side #24hourThumbsUp"
- If necessary, alert your close friends and family that you're taking a 24 hour phone detox and that they will need to get hold of you via other methods.
- If you're expecting important emails, set-up an automatic response message to notify the sender that you will get back to them in 24 hours.
- Some activities require you to contact your friends or family. We advise you to make a list of phone numbers (landline and mobile) as well as their home addresses.

- If you normally use your phone as an alarm clock – make another plan for tomorrow. Unless you can make a firm resolution to turn your phone off the *instant* you wake up.

Great! This next step is super important.

It is, of course, your Thumbs Up commitment. Repeat after me:

"I challenge myself to part with my smartphone for a full 24 hours. My thumbs will be free! Every time I'm tempted to use my smartphone, every time I'd normally be using it - I'll just do something awesome instead. In the REAL world!"

And so the adventure begins!

1. Locate your phone's power button.
2. This is a big moment for you. Take a deep breath. Count to three.
3. Press it.
4. Store your phone somewhere secure and out of sight. Or give it to someone you trust for safekeeping.

You've done it!

Possible side-effects may include:

- Fidgeting.
- Heightened awareness, amazing clarity and focus.
- Uncontrollable thumb twitching.
- Intense attraction to digital objects.
- The realization you're doing something most people are too scared to try, followed by the realization that this makes you awesome!

That's it! Turn the page and let's begin.

Chapter 1 – Rise and shine!

Ah! A new day. A very new day. You begin your 24 hour Thumbs Up challenge RIGHT NOW! I know you're probably craving to check your Facebook notifications but just bear with me, I have a stack of activities to kick-start the adventure.

So jump right out of bed – it's time to choose just ONE of the activities below. Don't think about it, just skim over them and go with your first impulse.

As soon as you have one, JUST DO IT!

If you dig it, and have enough time, just keep choosing and doing. Now go, go, go!

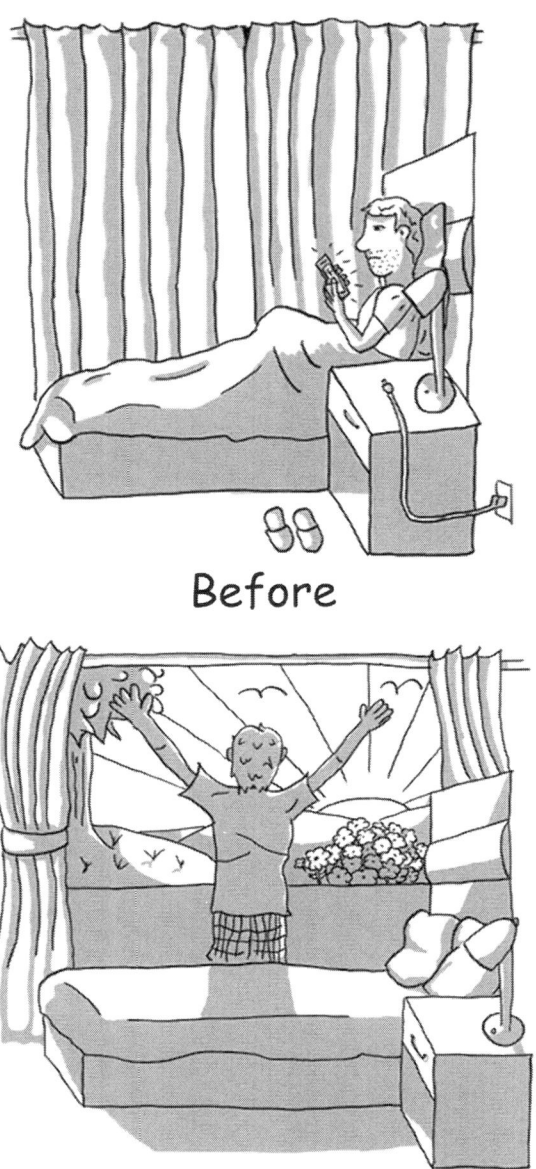

Before

After

Productivity

1. Cultivate a new routine! Do this immediately upon getting out of bed. Just do one or combine them into a super sequence!

   - Drink a full glass of water.

   - Do a quick yoga session – add a new move to your routine every day (the Sun Salutation is a great one to start with).

   - Smile at yourself in the mirror for 30 seconds. Remind yourself of everything that's going well in your life and think about all the things you have to be grateful for. Feels pretty good, right?

   - Commit to a home workout routine. No equipment? No excuses! Begin with simple bodyweight exercises. Or gather together heavy, awkwardly shaped items for a home gym. Try some exercises with your chair - use it for tricep dips or inclined push-ups. Deadlift that stack of books. Fill your backpack with heavy stuff and do fifty squats. Or, you know, you could actually go to the gym.

   - Perform a focused meditation on a specific topic. Think clearly and single-mindedly about only one topic for a period of time. Keep a notebook handy to jot down any ideas.

Now enjoy a kick ass day. Realize every day could start like this!

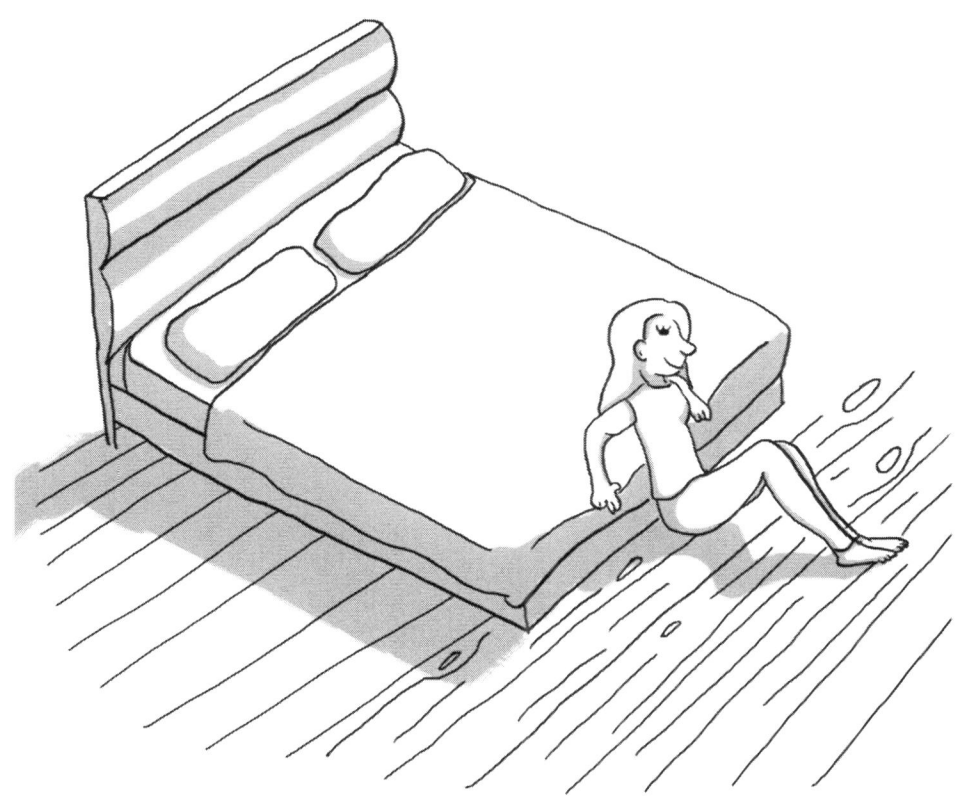

Do a simple morning exercise

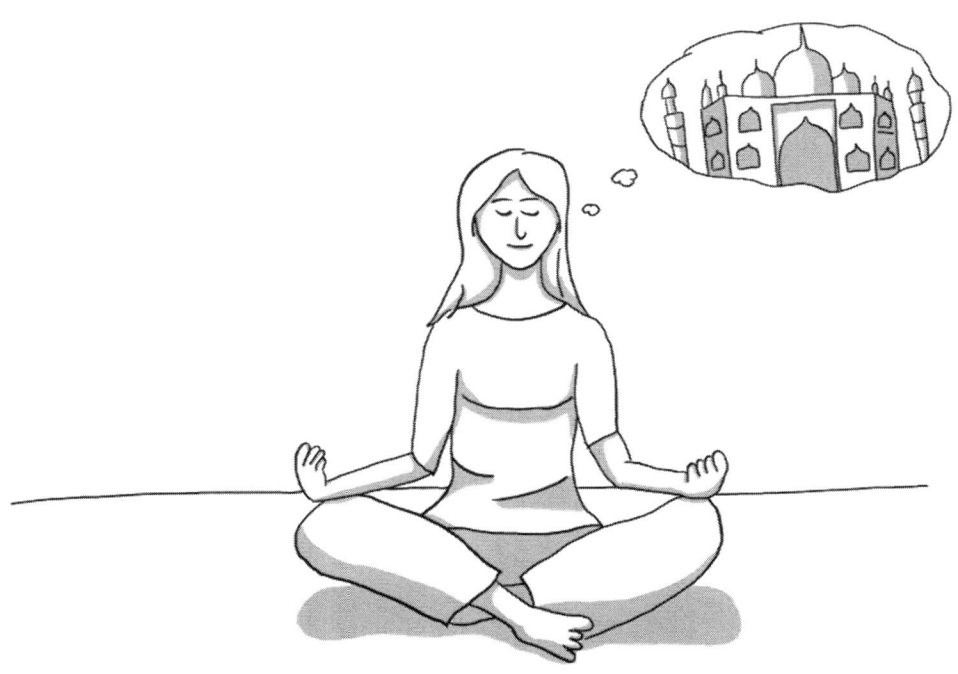

Meditate on a topic

2. Go outside to feel the weather before deciding what to wear. Or at least stick your head out of the window, breathe in a big helping of fresh air and take a moment to study the sky. Make your own weather prediction! What does that weather guy know, anyway?

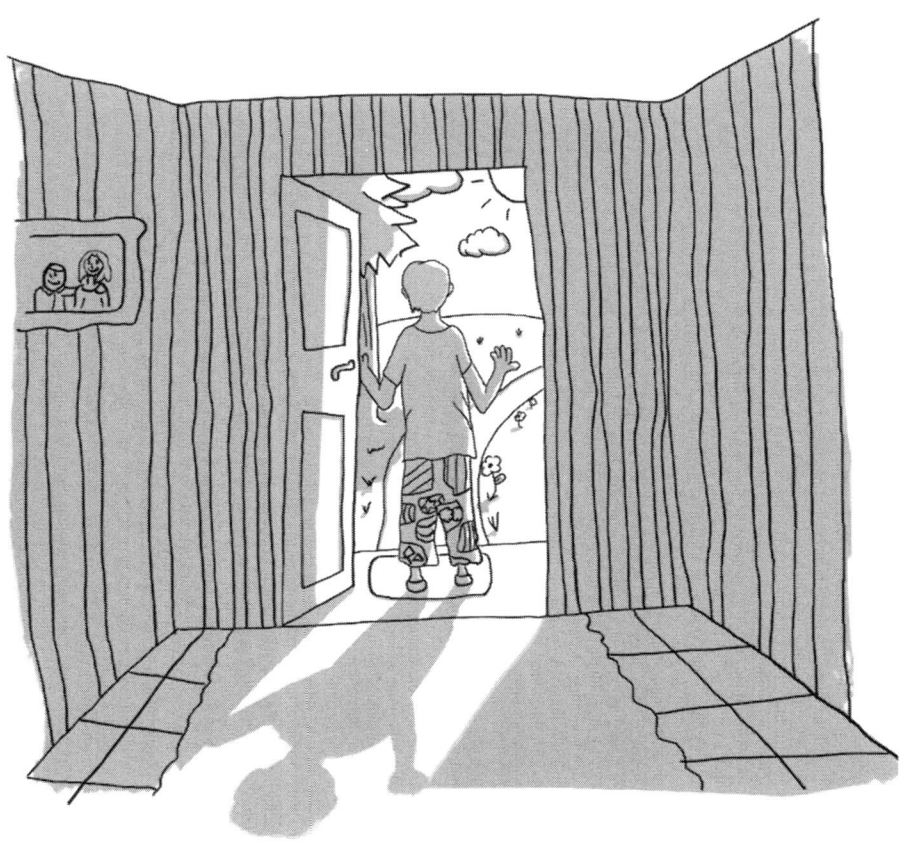

Feel the weather

3. Extra cleanliness! Extreme hygiene! Give your belly button a thorough scrubbing. Trim your nose and ear hairs. Treat and clean those nasty pimples and blackheads! To pop or not to pop, that is the question.

4. Grab a paper calendar to find out about important holidays and spend a few minutes memorizing the dates. While you're at it, pencil in all the birthdays and important dates you can remember. Use this as a daily memory exercise. You'll soon become a ninja at memory recall and never have to rely on your phone to replace your brain again!

5. Make a list of...
   - your aspirations.
   - a bunch of fun stuff to do.
   - 10 places you want to visit in the next 5 years.
   - all the household items you've neglected buying for far, far too long.

6. Instead of spending idle morning minutes Facebooking and YouTubing and skimming dating profiles, instead reclaim this time and spend it on YOURSELF. Look inwards instead of outwards. Give one of these a go!

- List the five things you admire most in others. Next to it list the five things you hate most in others. *Now realize you are looking into a mirror of the qualities you most like and dislike about yourself.* Whoa - mind blown!
- Conduct an interview with yourself: ask yourself what your favorite X, Y and Zs are, your favorite memories, and your ultimate sandwich toppings.
- Ask a close friend to describe both your most saintly virtues and your most annoying habits.
- Develop a new principle to live by.

7. Put a few minutes into some organizational wizardry!
   - Write out a shopping list! By hand! With a pen!
   - List what you want to get done by the end of the day. Order the list. Start doing these things and ticking them off. Give yourself deadlines and stick to them.
   - Schedule important appointments with your dentist, doctor, tutor, mentor, or your overwrought, neglected mother...
   - Organize your *real* desktop.

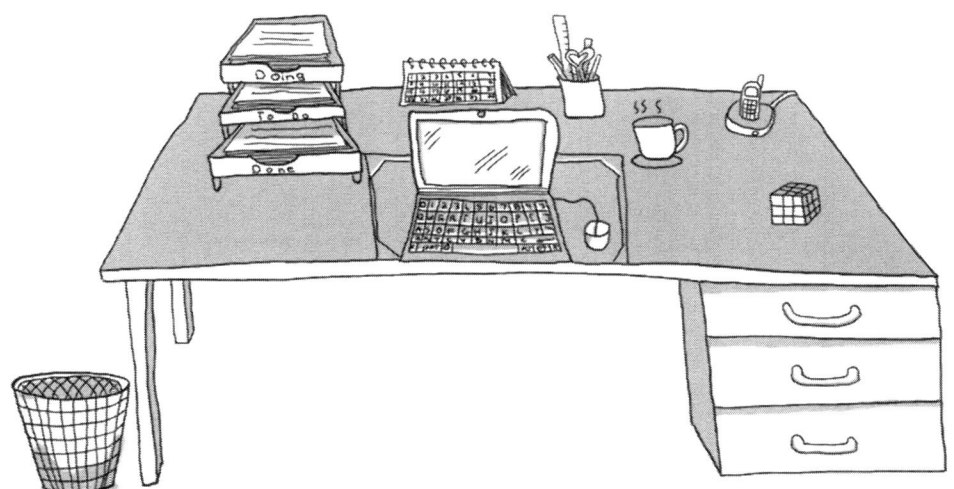

Organize REAL desktop

8. Cultivate a beneficial habit. Write it out on the bathroom mirror. Or stick it on the fridge. Or paste it on your door.

   - Stop doing irrelevant, superfluous activities.
   - Make a decision: "I will wake up 30 mins earlier tomorrow and in this time I will work single-mindedly on X" (one specific goal, project or skill). Set your alarm *now*.
   - Commit to remembering people's names when you first meet them. Treat it as a memory exercise. A good trick is associating crazy images or words with the sound/meaning of their first and last names.

9. Read the news from a *real* newspaper. How great is it to hear the rustle of the paper, to hold something bigger than your palm for a change!? Plus there is the novelty of getting your news from *one* source instead of scattered articles shared by all your random Facebook contacts...

10. Go grocery shopping at a farmer's market. Get some fresh, wholesome foods and cook an insanely healthy meal. Start the day off with an epic omelet packed with organic goodness. Whiz up a green smoothie.

11. Give your pets a bit of love! Groom them! Give them a quick bath. Put ribbons in their hair – no, not for Instagram, but just because they are your pets and you want to make *them* feel special.

12. Color code your keys.

Connection

1. Start your day with a commitment. Choose one of these and
    constantly remind yourself to practice it throughout the day.

    - Smile and be friendly to EVERYONE today, no matter what.
      You are going to make a bunch of other people smile in
      return, I promise. And in that moment you're connected.
      It's that easy.

    - DECIDE to be positive and hang around positive people
      until you go to bed tonight.

    - Honk and wave to random strangers on your way to work.
      You are going to get some priceless reactions.

    - Don't pass judgment (on yourself OR on others) for the
      entire day.

    - Don't compare yourself to anyone else AT ALL today!

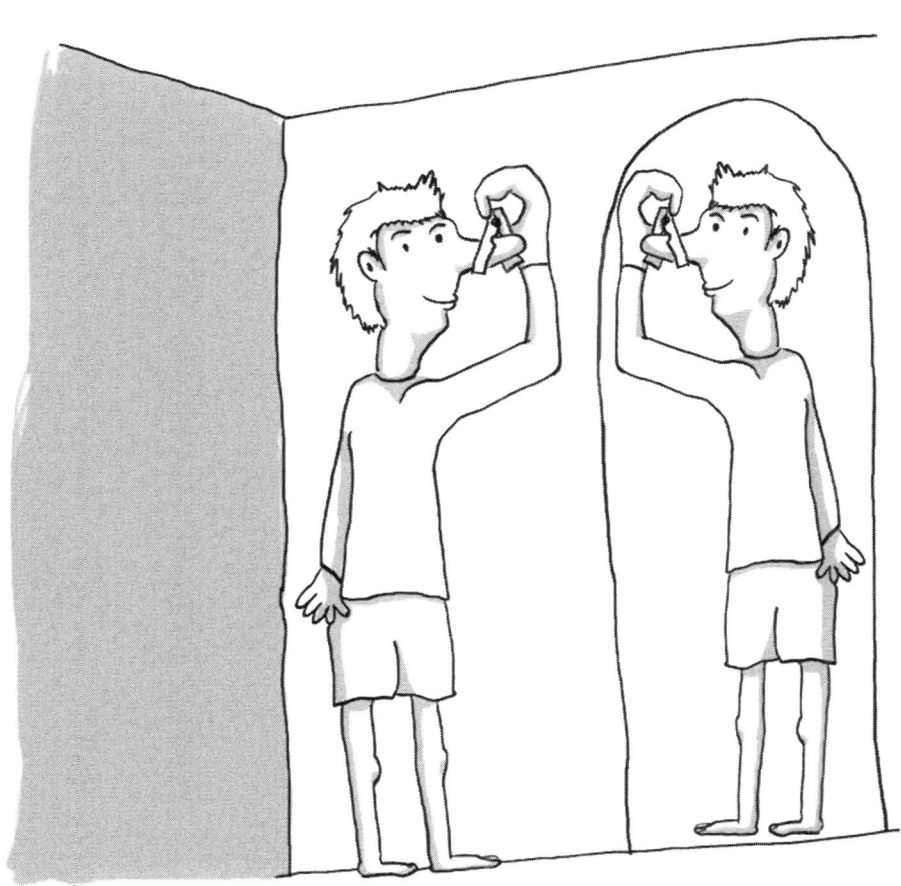

Don't judge

2. Spread the positivity! You'll feel AWESOME after you do one of these, and the feeling is guaranteed to linger, so try to get it done as early in the day as possible!

    - Smile at someone in the elevator.
    - Give up a grudge. Forgive and forget. For something small, or for something big (like that terrible person who took a bite out of your turkey sandwich). Forgive them in your own head, or actually go tell them face to face.
    - Buy food for a homeless guy. Take a moment to bask in the gratitude.
    - Help out someone in need. Be it a stranger, a friend, or a family member.
    - Share a taxi with a stranger. Chat. Split the fare (or offer to pay for your cab buddy and be that little bit more awesome).

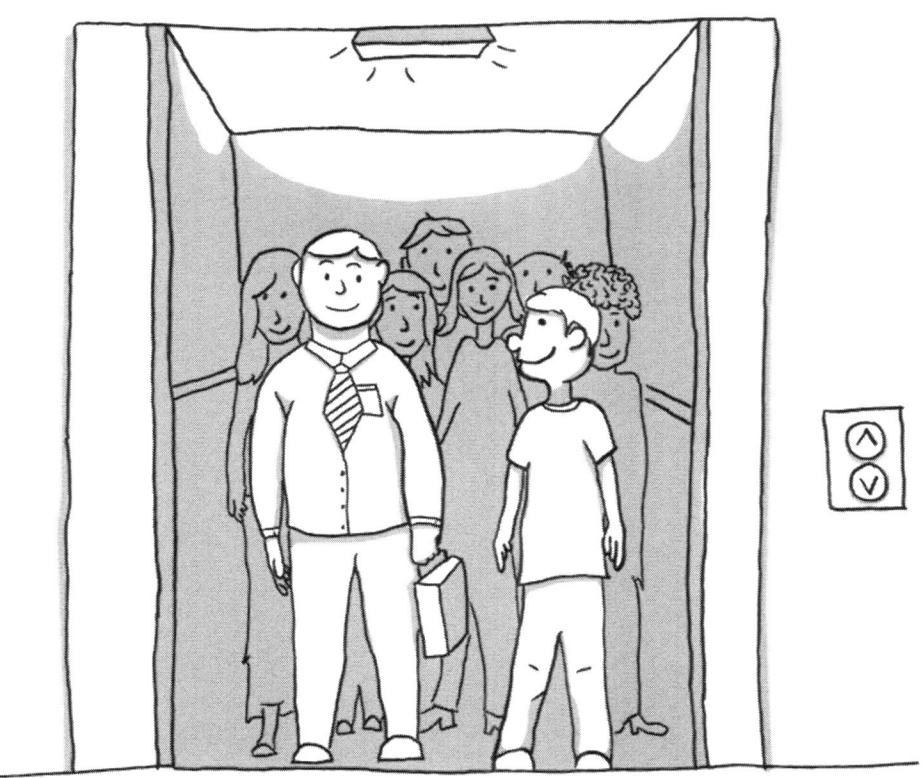

Smile at strangers

3. Use this super simple icebreaker to initiate a conversation with the first person you see today: ask a friend, family member or colleague what they dreamed about last night. Make sure you share *your* crazy dream about navigating the arctic on a whale you lassoed with rope you made from mermaid's hair.

4. Make the entire family a scrumptious breakfast. Or even just for your cat. Treat them!

5. Be observant. You're no longer staring at a tiny screen throughout the day, so make the conscious effort to notice the little things. Notice the samurai sword tattooed on your car pool buddy's arm, notice how your dentist's receptionist dyed her hair a different shade of mauve. Now make a point of commenting on what you've noticed. You don't have to start a life-changing conversation, just mention it in a way which shows you care. It's a chance to make the other person feel good.

6. Here are a few really 'out there' suggestions. These are pretty epic ways to put yourself in the shoes of someone living a life radically different from your own.

- Spend a period of time blindfolded to simulate what it would be like to lose your sight.
- Stick in some earplugs and spend some time in absolute silence. Carry out your day as usual with your sense of hearing impaired.
- Humble yourself. Become a beggar for a day.

The point of doing one of these is to further *connection* – so the next step is to *share* this experience. Inspire someone else to try this for themselves. Compare notes about it afterwards.

Entertainment

1. Stare at your own face in the mirror for a long time. Really study it. See what happens, notice your thoughts, see if you can spot a few things you haven't seen before. And make sure you spend time focusing on the bits you like best!

2. Stylize your facial hair. Or, if you're a lady, then just your hair. While you're at it why not dye it a darker shade of pale? Or deep crimson?

3. Smell the flowers. Close your eyes and breathe deep. If there are no flowers nearby – *make sure you find some today!* If there really are no flowers anywhere nearby it's time to flee. Throw some clothes into a backpack and get the hell out of there, dude!

4. Scream something for the entire world to hear. It doesn't matter what. Just scream, raw and primal like Dakota Fanning at her best. Or yell something profound like "I'm still alive!" or "I LOVE BANANAS!"
    The point is to not give a rat's ass for a moment. To feel that.

5. Picture and relive your happiest memories.

6. Watch your cat do silly things. Just watch. No video recording, no pictures, no trying to capture the antics in any place but your own memory. Heck, maybe even play with your cat! Now where is that ball of string...?

7. Listen to podcast. Listen to an audiobook. Set the tone for the day by filling your mind with new knowledge or inspiration.

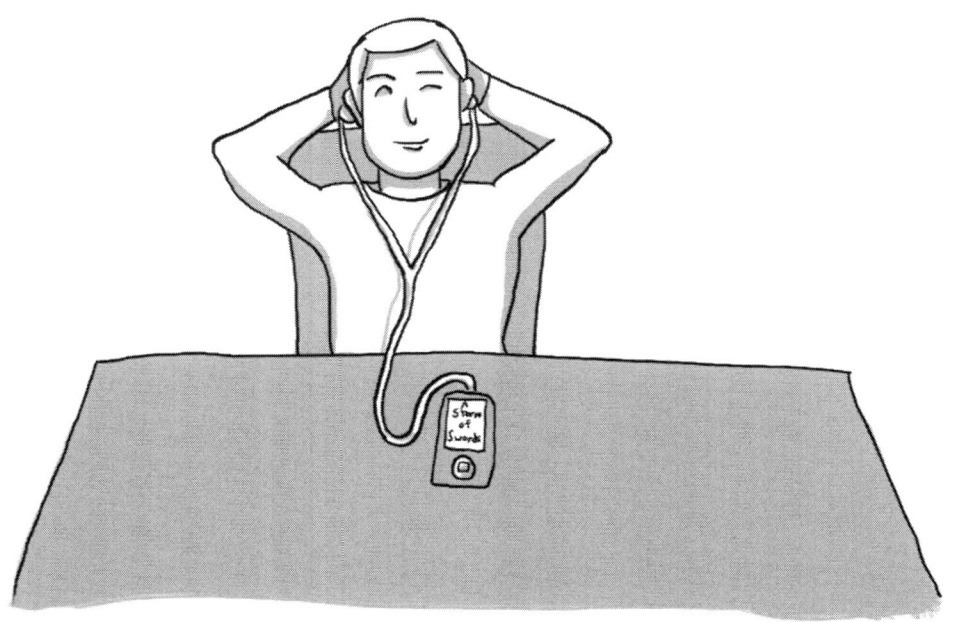

Listen to an audiobook

8. Skip everywhere instead of walking.

9. Practice the power of the voice.

   - Impersonate famous people or movie characters.

   - Adopt an accent for the whole day.

   - Talk really, r e a l l y, s l o w l y.

   - Speak absolute gobbledygook for a full minute of conversation.

   - Laugh out loud spontaneously.

   - Put the TV on mute and lip-synch your own dialogue.

   - Make up a (secret) language.

   - Read a story out loud. To yourself, or to anyone willing to listen.

   - Speak ye in yon Olden Day Prattle. Be grandiose, and verbose, and punctilious. Quote Shakespeare till you annoy people.

10. Grate butter on your toast instead of spreading it. Because - *why not?* Now apply this mindset to something else too, it's great. Instead of doubting a decision or an action just think *why not?* Then go do it.

11. Start trying to solve a Rubik's cube or do a crossword puzzle. No hints, tips, or tricks. Make this your morning project and keep at it every morning for a few minutes.

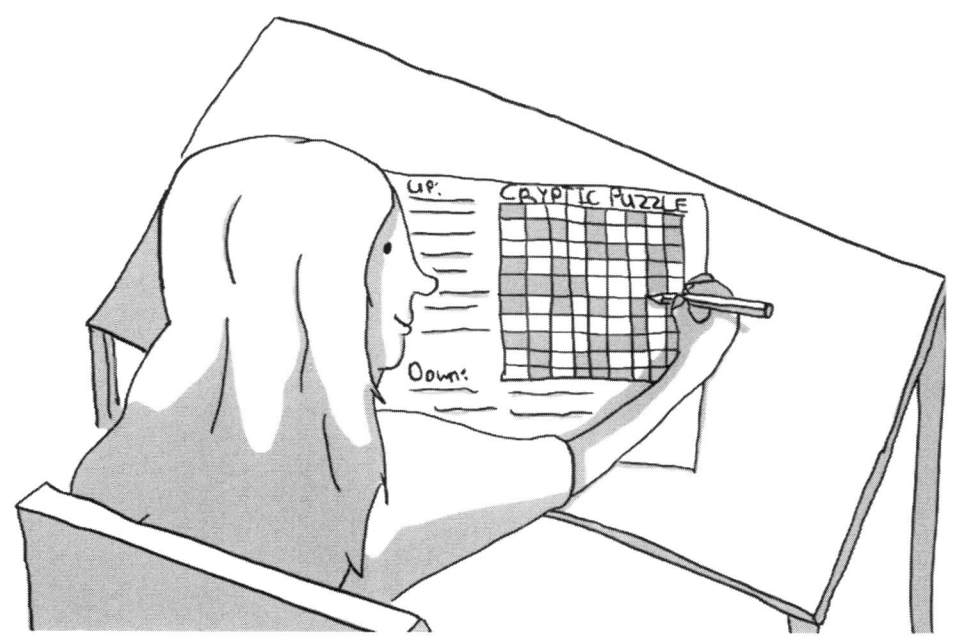

Do a crossword

12. Go for a hike.

    You won't be able to snap pictures with your phone along the way. You'll have to make your own memories. This means you'll have to sit down and take the time to really soak in that panorama from the top of the mountain.

    You'll experience the present moment and learn to linger in it. Because when you do move on you won't have a photo to remind you of what you experienced. And that's the point. When something catches your eye, a face-shaped boulder, say, or the toppled remnants of an ancient tree, you'll slow down, you'll trace the gnarled details in the bark with your eyes and really let it sink in because when you move on all you'll have are your memories.

13. Catch the sunrise if you can. Or else wake up early tomorrow and see it peak over the horizon.

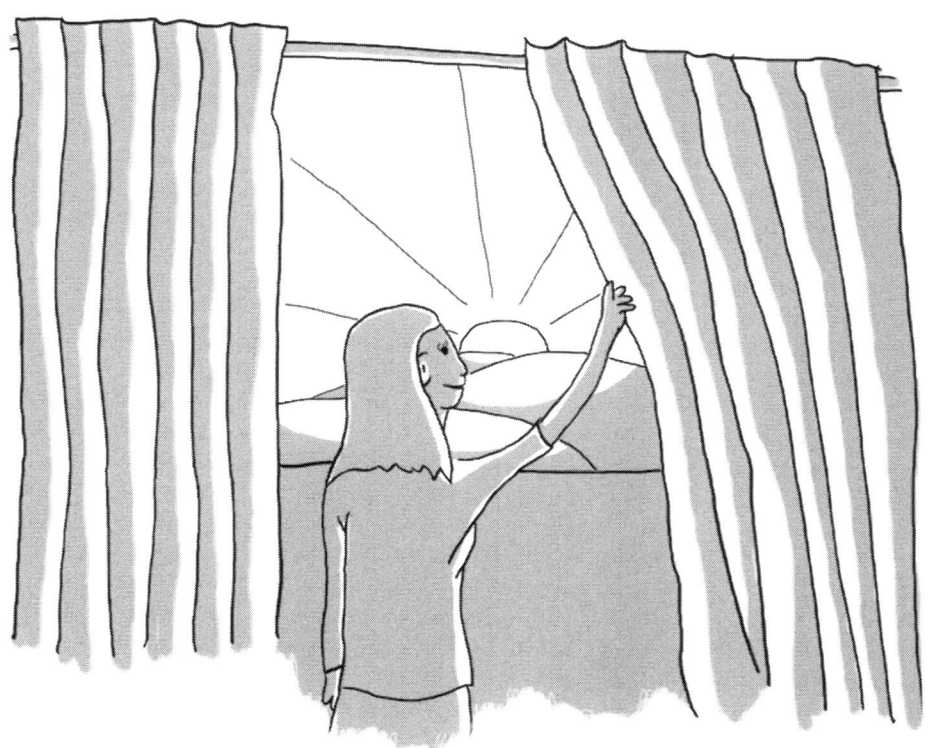

Catch the sunrise

Chapter 2 – Bettering the grind.

You're in the swing of things, you've left the house and begun work, school or running your errands. If you're super lucky, you have some free time right about *now*.

See which of the following activities you can accomplish wherever you happen to be, whenever you get the chance.

Because let's face it, you would otherwise just been flicking a few angry birds across a tiny blue sky. Now you can't, because you have chosen to part with your smartphone for a whole day. Like a boss. You've given yourself the opportunity for adventure instead. So use it! Right now!

YESNESS!

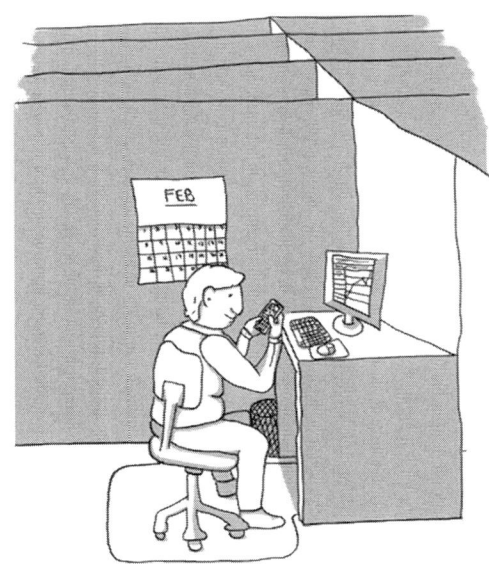

Before

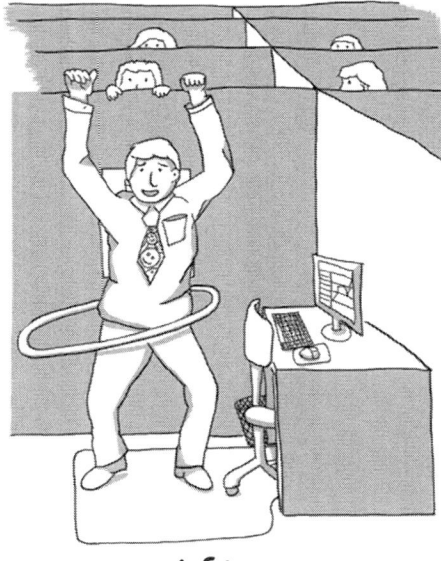

After

Connection

1. Dish out a single compliment. Later, find someone else and dish out another. Keep a tally. The point here is this: if you are actively trying to compliment someone you're finding and focusing on something positive in the other person. Whoa – that's way deep, bro!

2. High five everyone at the office. Or in the mall, or passersby on the street – transform a boulevard of broken dreams into a street of smiles. Corny? Sure. But highly effective. Trust me. Pro tip: you will *never* miss a high five if you watch the other person's elbow when you strike. True story. Test it. I'm serious.

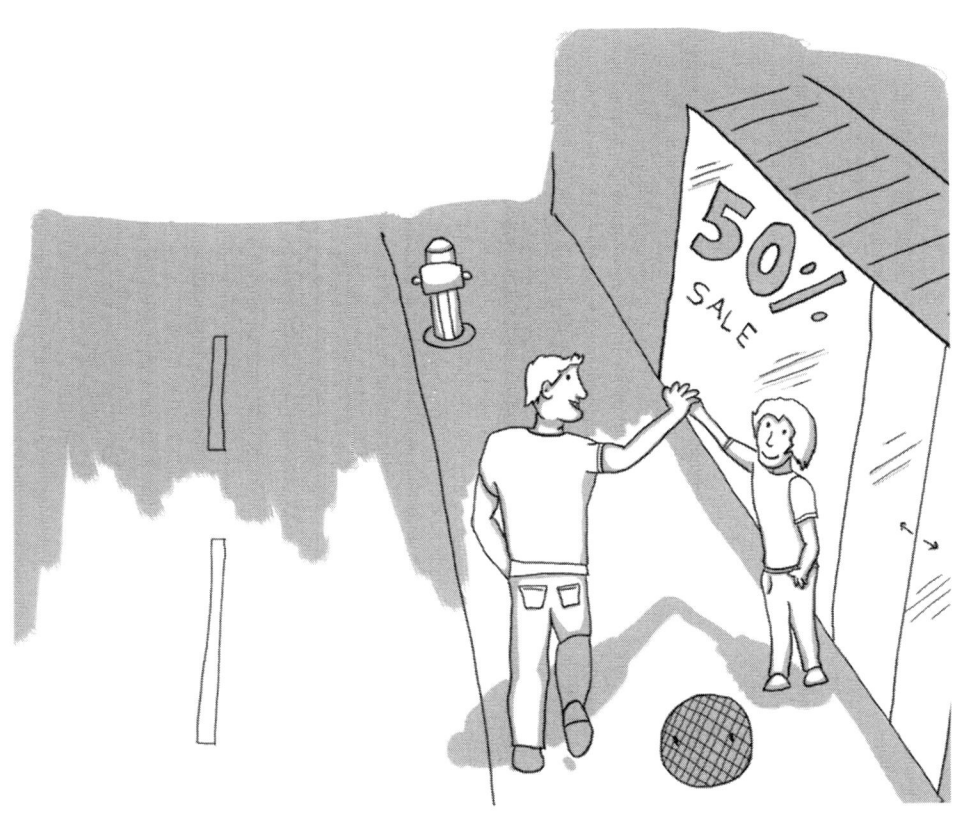

Hi-five people on the street

3. Tell a joke. Alternatively, try inventing one. For example...umm...you're on your own. Good luck!

4. Write a stage play and enact it with your most dramatic acquaintances. Okay, this one will take some time. But why not start now? Why not start with a short, humorous skit (perhaps ridiculing the most annoying thing about your boss...)

5. Plan out your own version of the Amazing Race.

6. Practice empathy. Actually listen to a friend talk to you, and draw out their true feelings, instead of just waiting for your turn to speak. Listen and try to find common ground or shared experiences so you can relate to them. Who knows, you might be able to offer some great advice you didn't know you had in you, or perhaps *receive* some insight into an area of your life you're frustrated with.

7. Begin correspondence with a pen pal via hand written letters. There's no school like the old school.

8. Have a DMC (deep, meaningful conversation).

9. Write a personalized message of gratitude to your parents/spouse/best friend. Post it to them, or go tell them in person (accompanied by a big hug).

10. Use a landline to cold-call someone you always wanted to get to know. It might be super awkward at first. It probably will be. Whatever. Power through it. Because why not? If you make an absolute ass of yourself, that's actually a *good* thing. Here's why – now you have an embarrassing story to share with someone else. And they will relate to it, and it will make them giggle, because everyone knows that awkward feeling when a conversation turns into a stuttering wreckage of insecurity. Sharing a story like that is a magical way to *ensure* connection with someone else. But hopefully the cold-call turns out just fine and you've made a new contact. I'm totally rooting for you! The point is that *either way you win.*

11. Stand up to someone you wouldn't normally stand up to. With words, not fists. Unless fists are necessary. And if they are, remember this: beneath Chuck Norris's beard is just another fist. I've seen it.

12. Write humorous responses to ads in the newspaper.

13. Ask someone knowledgeable for information instead of Googling.

- Talk to someone about *their* interests and learn about *their* world. Ask your grandmother about life before smartphones.

- Befriend someone who is an expert in their field. Get them to teach you something cool. Perhaps you can teach them something too, and if you can, do.

14. Network with people *without* using social media.

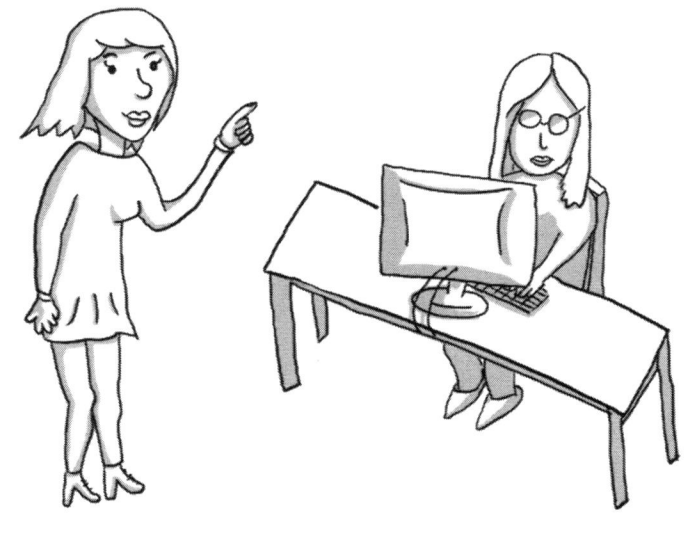

Ask someone instead of Googling

Productivity

1. Flip through a *real* dictionary and learn three new words. Study their etymology, try to pronounce them using phonetic symbols. Then immediately work them into the next few conversations you have.

2. Replace one cup of coffee/tea/juice/soda with one glass of water. You know, for your health and all that.

3. Search for addresses and phone numbers using an actual phone directory. Write out a list of emergency phone numbers keep them in your wallet. And stick them to the fridge. Why haven't you already done this!? Add a few of your closest friends' and relatives' numbers to the list for good measure. Memorize them. This could totally save your life.

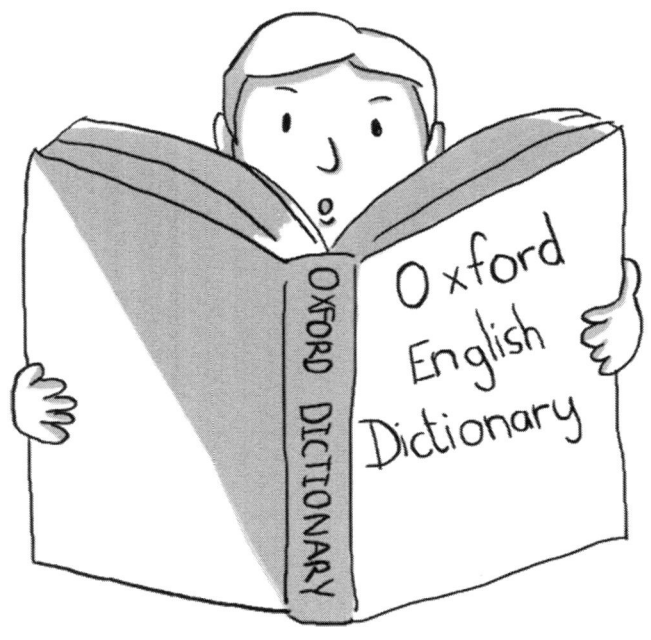

Use a dictionary

4. Sit down with pen and paper and do some serious planning. Clear everything from your immediate field of vision and focus only on a single idea. The point here is to free yourself of all distraction, to narrow your attention.

   - Jot out the character sketches for that novel you've always dreamed of writing but haven't started yet. Make this the start.

   - Plan your own YouTube channel, podcast or blog.

   - Compose a song.

   - Draft a campaign for a cause you care about - a charity perhaps, or an NGO, or a pet shelter. Put some energy into making the world a better place.

   - Come up with a crazy idea for a Kickstarter project.

   - Plan a road trip with your buddies from high school.

   - Or chart out an inner journey.

5. Snap your fingers as if you just had a great idea and see if you actually get one.

6. Create a *real-life* Pinterest board! Bonus: you get to press with thumb tacks into a cork board. YESNESS!

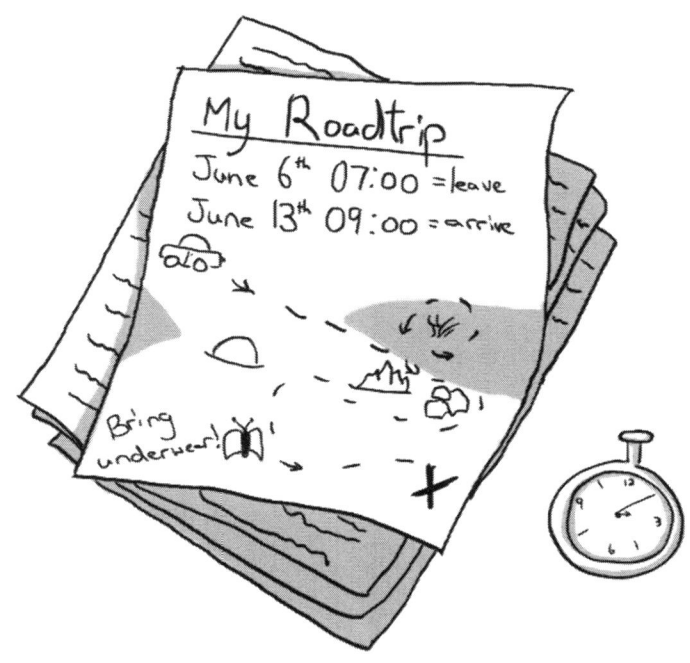

Do some serious planning on paper

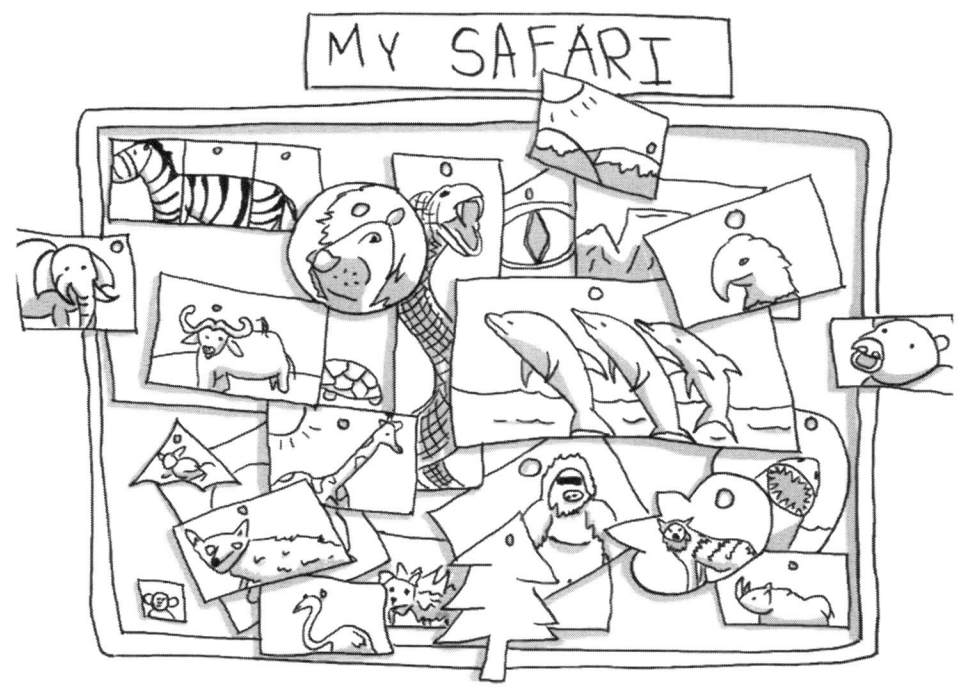

Create a REAL Pinterest board

7. Invent something to make your life easier. You know, like Steve Jobs did. Or just a better way to store your sandwiches. You choose.

8. Do just *one* thing you have been putting off. Do it. Right now. Seriously. You know what it is. It's the thing that's popping into your mind right now. Do it. Now. I'm serious, just go do it. Okay, I know I played a dirty trick on you, because by now that thing is looping in your mind like a bad song. You probably hate me. That's fine.
SO JUST GO DO IT!
And then it will be done. And you will be so grateful. You'll still hate me, but you'll be super pleased with yourself. And I can live with that.

9. Find a niche in a market. Generate a strategy to exploit it! Become a millionaire! Yup, it might actually be that easy. You might just get an idea that changes the world as we know it in 3, 2, 1...

10. Polish and update your CV.

11. Identify and stop a single bad habit.

    This is a tricky one, but it can be broken down into a few simple steps. It's a process of rewiring your brain, of *replacing* the habit with a new automatic behavior.

    - First, identify the habit itself, the actual behavior (turning on the TV as soon as you walk into the house).
    - Second, identify the cause/environment/stimulus that triggers this habit (walking into the house).
    - Third, identify the reward this habit gives you (the joys of procrastination).
    - The hard part: now you need to either avoid the cause of the habit or do something else instead, while still offering yourself a reward for the new, more constructive habit.

    Yes, you'll probably slip back into your old behavior a few times. That's just how it goes. But gradually you *will* overwrite the old neural pathways and finally be rid of that pesky old habit. And then you can totally pat yourself on the back.

12. Impart one of your skills to a newbie. Even something as mundane (to you) as teaching someone how to staple pages properly, or write an essay, or drive a tractor.

13. Brainstorm some ways you could generate passive income.

14. Become famous. How? That's up to you.

15. The Buddy System.

- Break down one of your goals into bite-size, actionable steps.
- Find friends and family members who you can share these steps with and ask them to hold you accountable for working towards achieving them.
- Ask them to check in on you regularly. Ask them to be hard on you if you're not delivering on your promise to them.

Entertainment

1. Here are a few silly ones. Silly, sure, but truly entertaining.

   - Lick your tongue. No, wait...that's not right...
     What I *meant* to say was kiss your elbow. Lick your nose.
     Make extremely loud fart sounds with your armpit.
   - Make a ridiculous number of photocopies.
   - Try moving things with your mind.
   - Any time someone asks you something, respond with "Do you want fries with that?"
   - Spin manically in your swivel chair.
   - Chew gum loudly. Blow bubbles. Be like that guy on the bus everyone is secretly peeved at. Purely for your own entertainment.
   - Stare at people until they break eye-contact. Practice your game face. Keep a tally: ME vs. EVERYONE ELSE. Gloat over every victory. Resolve to be more badass after every defeat.
   - Send an email to the entire staff: "If anyone needs me, I'll be conducting some urgent business in the bathroom."
   - Tell someone who is sitting quietly that they are being extremely noisy and could they please quiet down thank you very much.

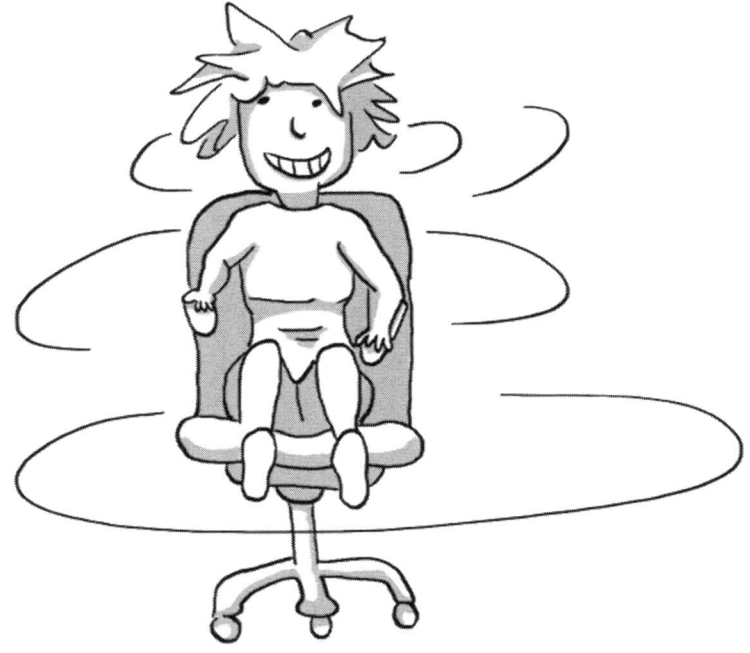

Spin manically on swivel chair

2. Think of a good memory and relive it.

3. Get some blood flowing!

   - Start dancing spontaneously without any music.

   - Finally master rubbing your belly while patting your head at the same time.

   - Crack your knuckles and other joints. Roll your shoulders. De-stress.

   - Dust off that old hula-hoop and swivel those hips! Yes, right there in the office. *Why not!?*

   - Land a back-flip.

   - Spin until you're dizzy (then try and walk in a straight line), do cartwheels, breakdance, get awesome at handstands – or headstands.

Chapter 3 – Break time. But not really...

You're already halfway! You've barely thought about your phone. But now...now you do. You miss it. You want to touch it. You want to let your brain turn into the unproductive mush which sloshes around between the ears of zombies...

This chapter is aimed at those stretches of time you'd normally spend zombifying yourself doing blah-blah swipey-swipe on your smartphone.

BUT NOT TODAY!

Today you will transform these zombie minutes into sheer

awesomeness! Instead you'll get energized, you'll actually DO something. You'll do it with verve, with pizzazz, and your efforts will cause you to GROW AN EXTRA BRAIN!

Ironically, this will make you more appealing to the zombies...

No worries though. You'll be so full of energy they'll never be able to catch you.

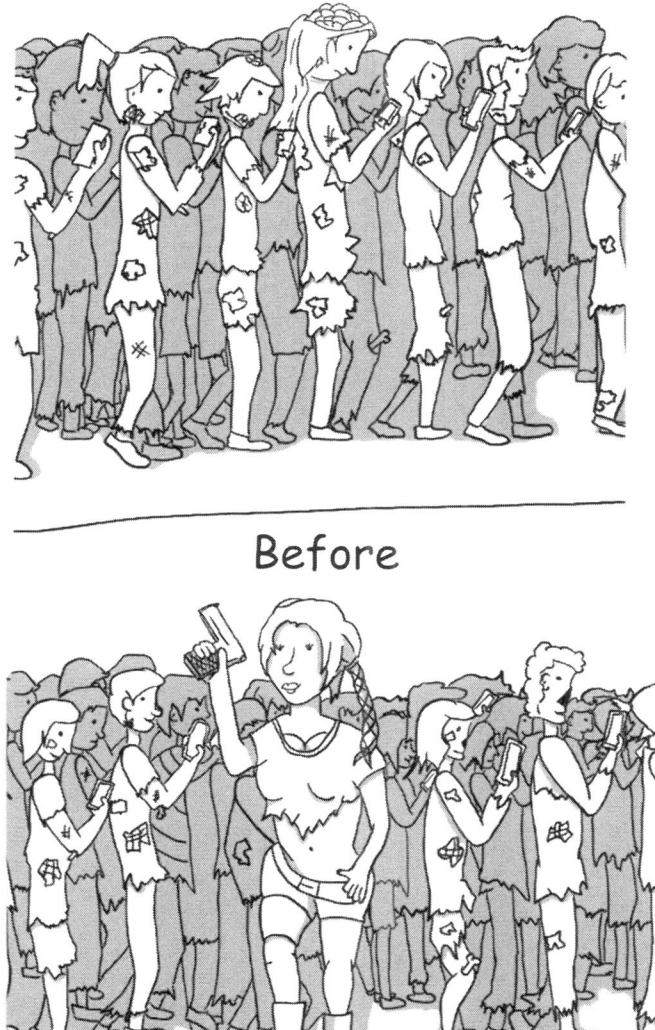

Before

After

Entertainment

1. You're still in the office. You feel like some shenanigans.

   - Grab a cloth and a spray bottle of cleaning agent. Then follow a colleague around like a ninja. Spray everything they touch and vigorously rub it clean. Pretend like they are spreading awful dirt and contamination.

   - Secretly switch the coffee to decaf and see if anyone notices...

   - Round up the most energetic people and have a three legged race down the hallway!

   - Ask your co-workers mysterious questions and write down their answers in a notebook. Mutter something about "psychological profiles."

   - Acquire chalk. Use it to chalk out a four-square court in the parking lot. Or hopscotch. Or scribble transient poetry between the parking spaces. Or spread chalk messages of hope and positivity. Or just doodle...

   - Play musical chairs and feel like kids again.

2. Count the number of cars/tourists/planes/buffalo that pass by (in a minute).

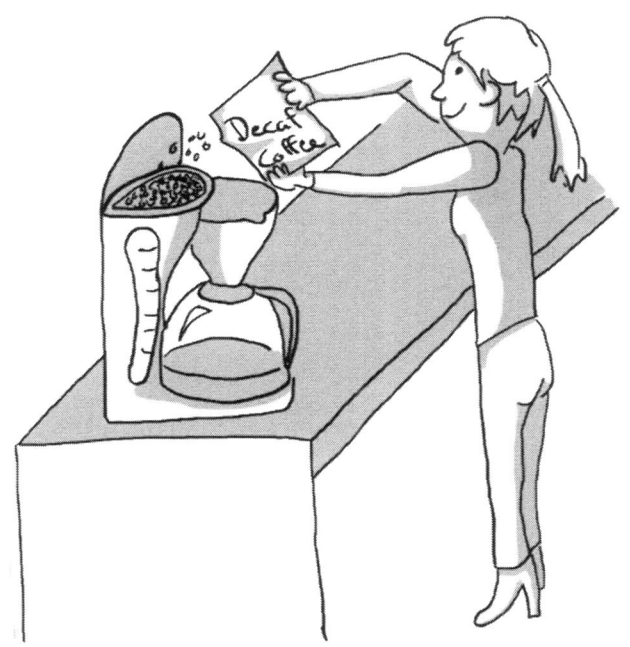

Switch office coffee to decaf

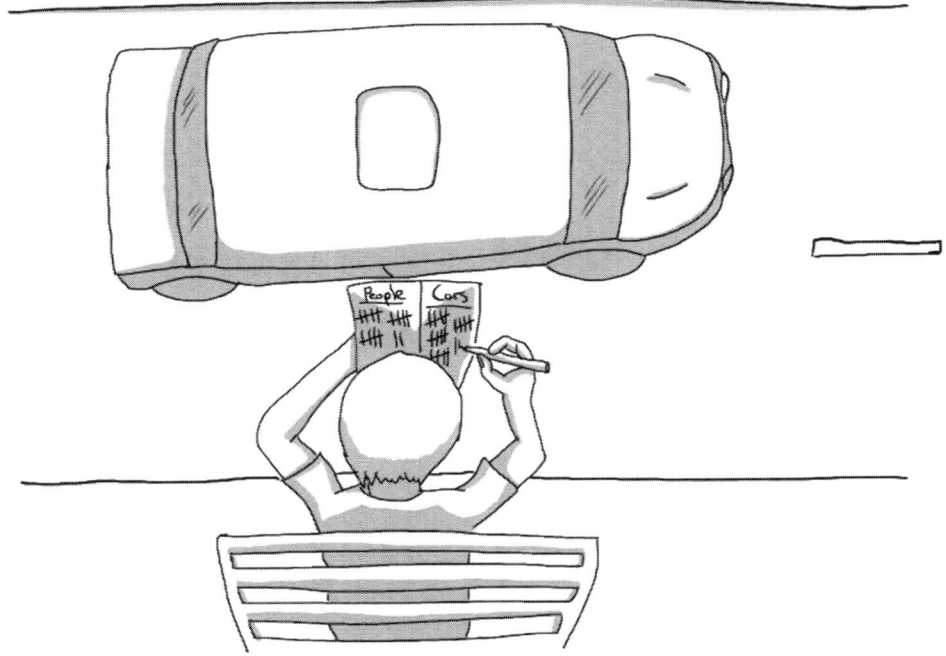

Observe people/cars that pass by

3. Nah. You're sick of being cooped up. So leave!

- Meander through an art gallery, but don't take it seriously. People watch, poke fun at the more ridiculous abstract pieces, laugh at the postmodern, and annoy the staff by being just a little too loud with your remarks.

- Dish out free hugs - go hug a stranger as if you know and love them. Just don't get arrested. Pick your targets wisely!

- Read real books! Go to the library and skim through a whole bunch of titles before choosing a select few. Savor each word. Why not make a dent in the 'Top 100 Books of All Time' list?

- Take a nap. No alarm. Give yourself permission to wake up whenever you do.

- Relax outside. Get high on life. Preferably in a hammock.

- Have your fortune guessed at by a palm reader. Why not tempt fate and try to read the palm reader's palm?

- Take up bug collecting, or study the little guys under a magnifying glass. Try to catch a lizard by the tail.

- Be inappropriately noisy in a public place.

- Break a world record for something – or set the benchmark for something which hasn't yet been attempted!

- Buy a donut and complain: "There's a hole in it."

- Build a house of cards. Experience just how fleeting and fragile it is precisely because you *can't* snap a picture of it on your phone. When it topples it is gone for good, there will be no evidence of your achievement. This is an experience worth having.

- Go on a quest to find a payphone. Once you've found it, call up a friend and explain you have completed your quest. Ask what you should go do next.

- Spend some time in an actual music store thumbing through the albums. Pick out a few based purely on the album art. Listen to them. Or ask that trendy staff member with the Mohawk and the tongue ring to recommend something totally obscure. Broaden your musical boundaries.

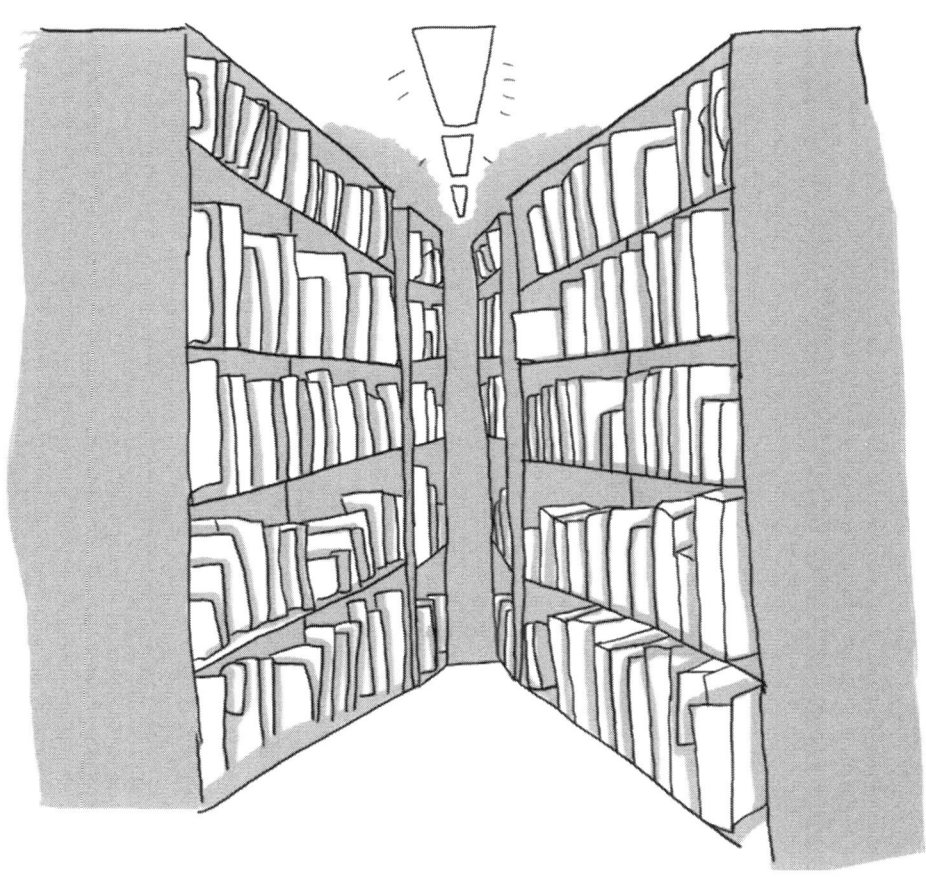

Visit the library

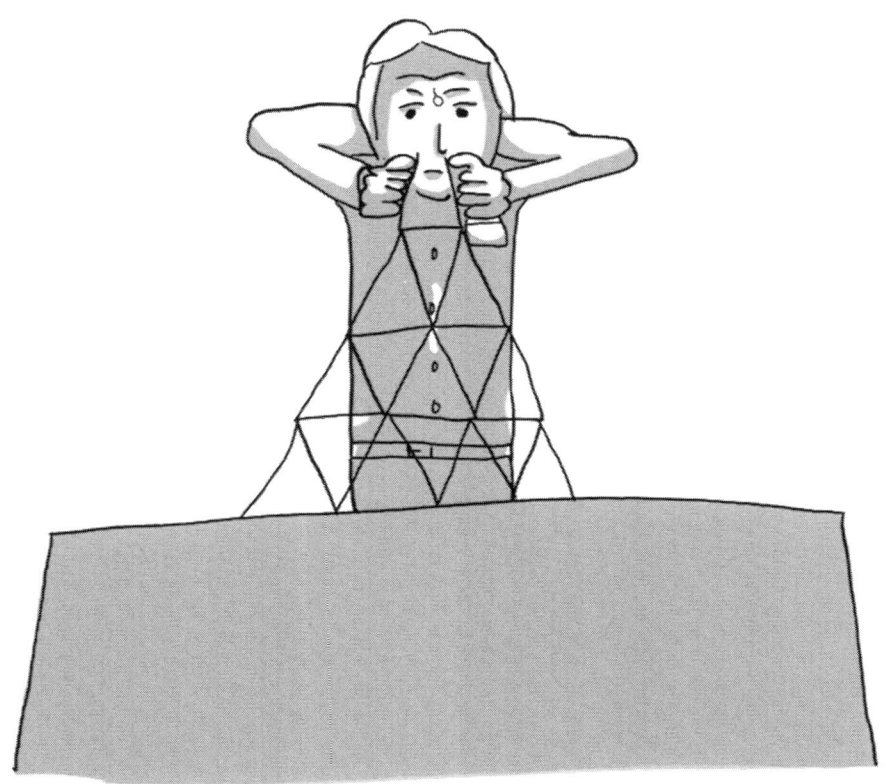

Build a house of cards

Connection

1. Start something which could become an office tradition!

   - Have a debating session. Divide up into teams. Pick an insanely controversial topic. Select a panel of judges.

   - Have a rap battle. Rhyme your own rhymes. Or plagiarize from the masters, yo.

   - Have a bring 'n share picnic on the office floor. With blankets and baskets and the whole shebang.

   - Initiate a food fight!

   - Hold an office auction for the best swivel chair.

   - Plan an office lottery to hand out those unpleasant duties/responsibilities.

   - Conduct weekly blind tastings. Train your tongue, hone your nose, create an elaborate system of awards for the best blind tasters. Also invent an extensive set of comical punishments for the losing team.

   - Host a Mad Hatter themed tea party. Make sure there is an abundance of cupcakes.

2. Share something you have. Whether it be as easy as a radiant smile, or as taxing as half your bar of chocolate - or as profound as giving away your spare paper clips...

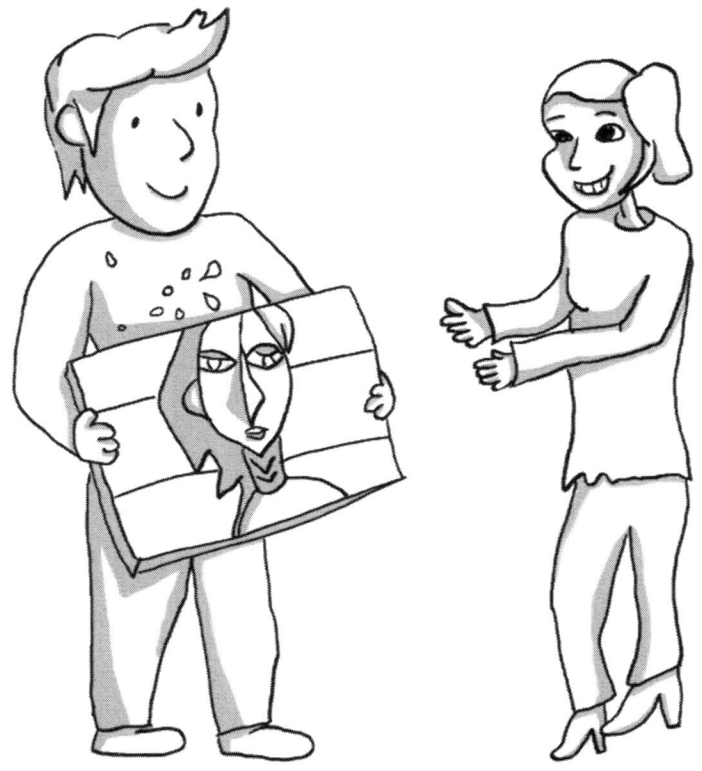

Share something with someone

3. Explain something you've just learned to a friend or a colleague. Notice how you now know this thing much more deeply. You're not only teaching them, you're also teaching yourself by actively thinking about it and trying to convey the information clearly and concisely. Do this regularly. This is also a great way to generate conversation topics.

4. Start a game of 'Charades' or 'Who Am I' or 'I Spy (With My Little Eye).' Because everybody could do with a little more light-hearted funsies.

5. Post a letter/card/photo to a distant relative or an estranged friend.

6. Talk to someone you're unstoppably attracted to. Just go do it. Start by saying "Hi." It really is that simple.

7. Go donate blood. You are literally saving someone's life by doing this.

Productivity

1. Memorize *deep* lines of poetry. Not only are you training your brain, you can totally use these lines to impress the ladies...

2. Make a thorough evaluation of your time management. How are you spending your time, and on what? How much time are you saving by not having access to a smartphone? Also, notice how you can stay focused for longer without constantly being distracted by beeps and buzzes. Your attention span is improving.

3. Enter yourself for a half-marathon. Pay the entrance fee. Now you're committed. Begin your slow but steady training schedule to prepare for the race. Why not start with a 1 mile run right now?

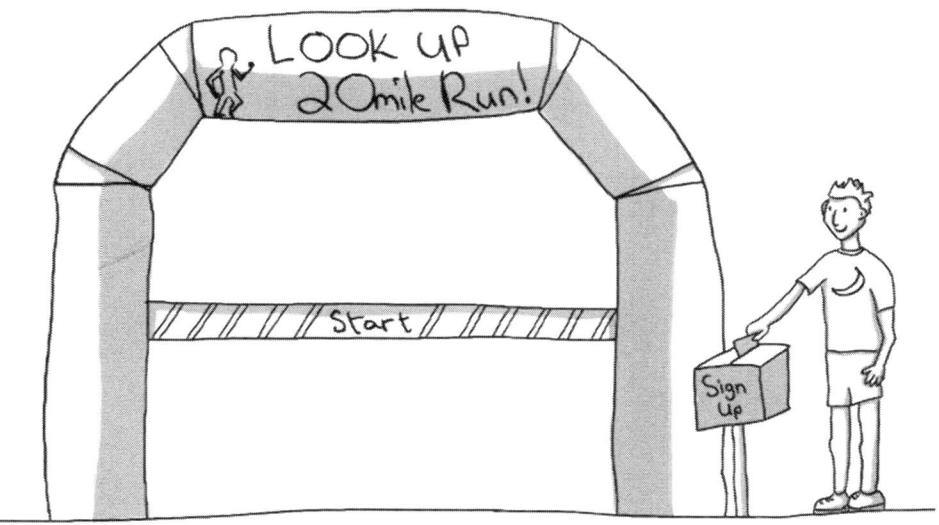

Enter yourself in a marathon

4. Give your employer a recommendation for an employee who is doing stellar work.

5. Start teaching an informal 20 minute crash course on something you're skilled at, whether it be work related or an absolute beginner's ukulele session for the other aspiring bards in the office.

6. Partner up with someone who shares a mutual interest and begin working on a side project.

7. Get as many of your daily chores, errands or tasks done RIGHT NOW so that you free up some time and energy for later on in the day.
   - Be prepared. Buy spares: light bulbs, batteries, candles, matches, cleaning materials, etc. You'll be so happy with yourself when you need one of these items and there it is!
   - Stock up on stationery.
   - Buy new underwear. Seriously. That old pair of...no, really, it's time.
   - Put together an "Apocalypse Survival Kit." This is a great excuse to stock up on canned tuna.

- Give some solid, constructive feedback to the manager of a store.

8. Memorize emergency phone numbers. Learn a new phone number every day. Train your brain.

9. Prepare gifts for birthdays or special holidays *now*. Instead of putting it off like you always do.
   Spend some time thinking about something awesome to get for the people in your life. Something truly meaningful, something they will actually use regularly or get real value from. No, not a box of chocolates. Dig deep. Make the effort. Or why not try to *make* some gifts for a change? Even a humble handmade card shows you have put care and effort into your gift.

10. Start eating more veggies. Vegetables, obviously, not vegetarians. OK, terrible joke. But do it. For real. It's good for you.

11. Try cubicle yoga. Use this down time to relax and loosen up after the demands of the morning.

Get a head start on your gift list

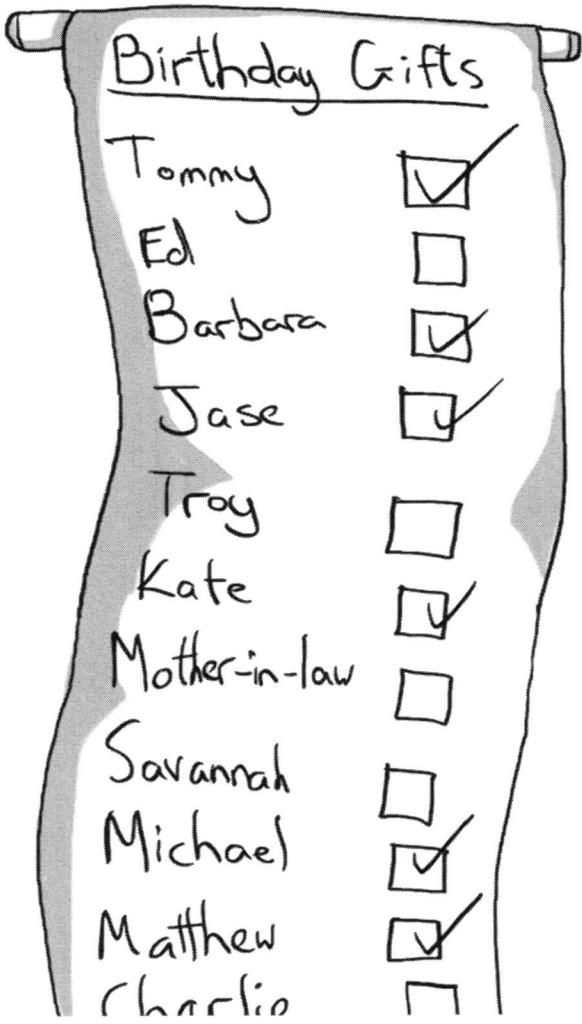

Chapter 4 – Right back at it!

Break time is over and now you're hard at work again. Except not really. You find you have free time because you've been so productive today. Good for you! But what to *do* with this time?

Every time you feel the urge to grab your smartphone – well, you can't, because you're Thumbs Up! Instead, dive right into another activity.

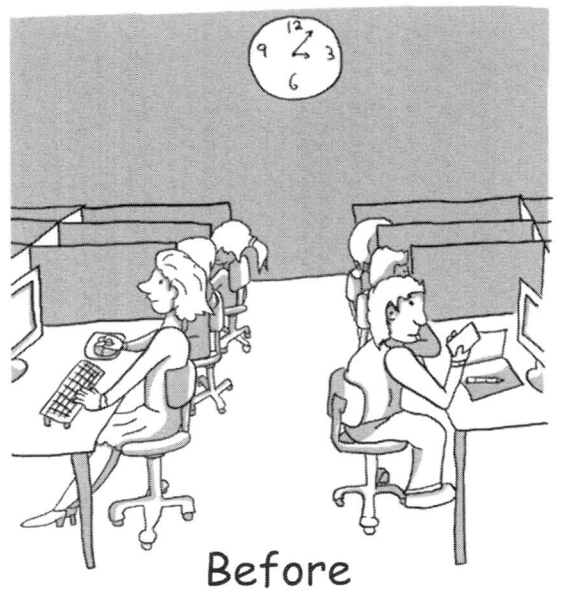

Before

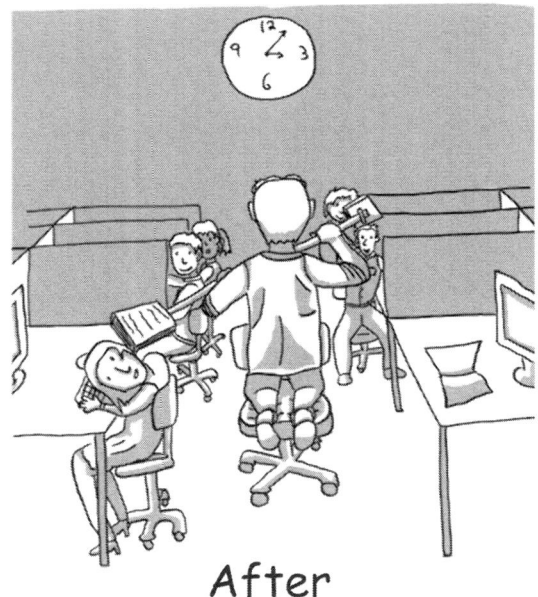

After

Connection

1. Plan a long holiday. Or even just a weekend escape. Camping. Fishing. A Sunday at the spa.

2. Initiate an epic game of broken telephone throughout the entire office. Be wildly inappropriate with your suggestive whispers.

3. Call someone you've been nervous to speak to.

4. Just ask. Ask for assistance with a difficult task, ask for help with a project you're struggling with, or ask someone to show you how to use the full range of features on the new espresso machine.

5. Tell stories.
   - That epic one about the time you were locked in your roommate's closet overnight.
   - Invent a new urban legend and begin spreading it.
   - Share an embarrassing moment you've never told your friends about.

- Create a group narrative masterpiece. Begin by choosing a Genre, a Time Period, a Setting, a Crisis and a Quirky Protagonist. Then take turns coming up with the next sentence in the story. You know, like that game you played with your family in the car on those long road trips when you were seven. It's still fun. For reals.

Productivity

1. Study a real map and learn the layout of a city, its area names and their relationship to each other. Memorize a few street names and commit some routes to memory so that you will be able to navigate a certain area without the use of Google Maps. Then get out there and test your newfound navigational wizardry!

2. Read up on a subject you know little about - no internet! Buy a book or a magazine on an unfamiliar topic. Spend some time expanding your mind and challenging your preconceptions. Expand your general knowledge.

3. Conduct your own experiments; come to your own conclusions. Be your own search engine.

4. Start learning a new skill:
   - Learn how to moonwalk, or how to fold origami.
   - Learn about finance and entrepreneurship.
   - Learn to program/code/hack.
   - Learn how to Photoshop – or just how to doodle in Paint.
   - Learn magic - or sign language.

- Learn exotic animal noises! Or Morse Code!

- Or finally learn how to build a website for that project you have been keeping on the back burner for months now...

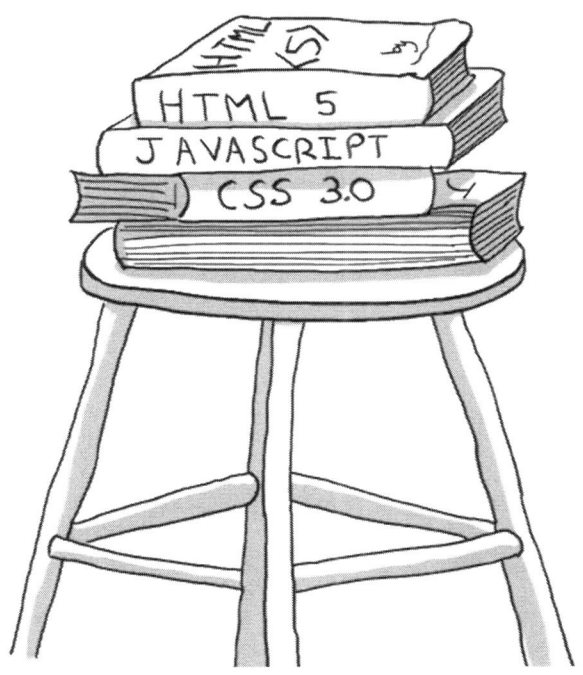

Learn to build a website

5. Study further in your favorite area of interest. Start by reading a super thick book.

6. Write a heartfelt, pen & ink love note. Seal it with a kiss, fold it with a smile, and post it to you-know-who.
   Or just write a good old-fashioned pen & ink letter to your grandma. They love getting those. What's all this e-mail nonsense? What is the world coming to!?

7. Find yourself a mentor – or better yet, begin to mentor someone else.

8. Reread an important document or article or essay.

9. *Reread an important document or article or essay!*

10. Brainstorm ideas for a business venture.

11. Do your taxes early this year.

12. Try to improve on something you already do well.

13. Satisfied with this job? Maybe it's time to apply for a new one…

Entertainment

1. Observe people. Laugh quietly to yourself at their silly behavior, or gossip furtively with a partner in crime.

2. Day dream. Go on an imaginative adventure. Construct an elaborate fantasy world in your head, a place populated with impossible people and home to inanimate animals. Push your mind to the limit. Play with possibility.

3. Watch a music video (and learn the dance). Perform it in your cubicle. Wave your hands in the air like you just don't care. Get your booty up on the desk.

4. An indoor treasure hunt! An outdoor treasure hunt! AN INDOOR AND OUTDOOR TREASURE HUNT! Mind. Blown.

5. Call up your mom and tell her you can't talk to her right now. Then hang up.

6. More office shenanigans!

- Write out messages and fold them into paper airplanes. Land them expertly onto the cluttered runways of your colleagues' desks.

- Get everyone in the office to form rowboat teams on their wheeled chairs. Race each other down the corridors and around the desks. Collide into stuff. Curse like pirates.

- Call yourself over the intercom. Make no attempt at disguising your voice.

- Put a trashcan on your desk. Print out a big, bold label "IN" and attach it to the trashcan.

- Play dead.

- Get bubblewrap. This achievement alone is awesome. Next: pop it. No - wait! Line the floor with it and jump on it. Bubblewrap hopscotch! No, wait wait wait! Wrap it around yourself till you resemble a plastic mummy and then roll around on the floor popping like crazy.

- Float a helium balloon to the ceiling and then try to get it down by shooting staples at it.

- Create finger characters by scribbling faces on your fingers. Give them vibrant personalities. Allow them to assume parts of your psyche and interact with each other.

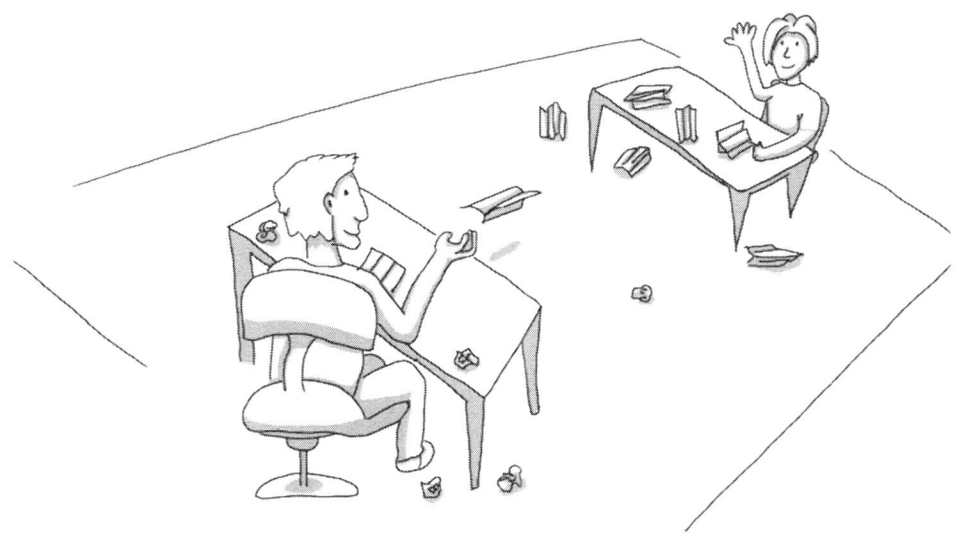

Write and fly messages to colleagues

Chapter 5 – Up, up and away. It's freedom time!

Work's over, school's out and the major obligations of the day are taken care of.

You've started feeling the benefits of your smartphone detox already, you're fired up by the activities you've already completed.

The time for true adventure begins now. You can do whatever you want, you get to choose from ANY of these epic activities.

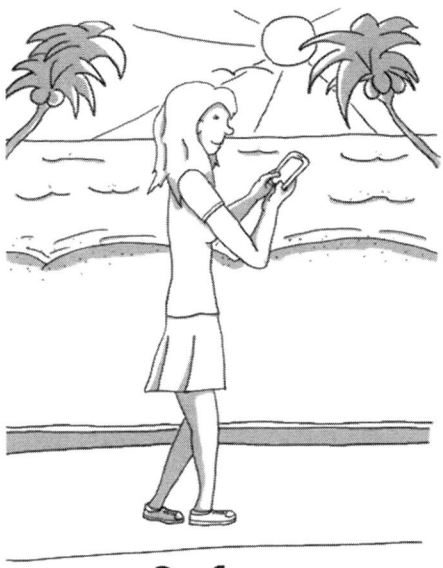

Before

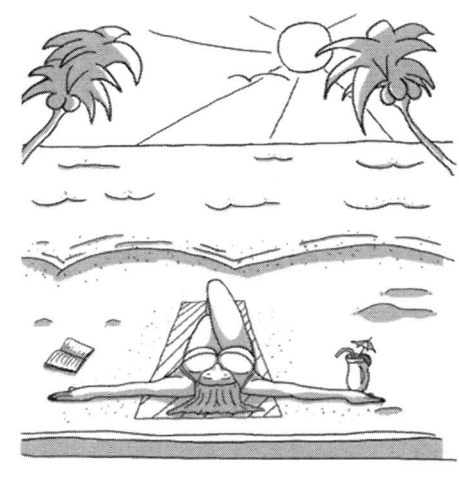

After

Connection

1. Go for Happy Hour. Alternatively, have Happy Hour in the office. Preferably inform your boss.

2. Rock out at a band jam session.

3. Get sporty!
   - Challenge your buddies to a fitness/strength competition. Cultivate the will to dominate and embarrass your friends with your insane calf raises!
   - What about an Extreme Household Object Weightlifting Elimination Challenge?
   - Get down to the beach and kick the soccer ball around, throw the Frisbee, invite strangers to join your game of French Cricket.
   - Join a social sports club. Become pro at ping-pong.
   - Brainstorm, invent and play a trial version of a new game based on the materials and environment you happen to be in right now. Come up with elaborate and unnecessary rules. Give it an outrageous scoring system.

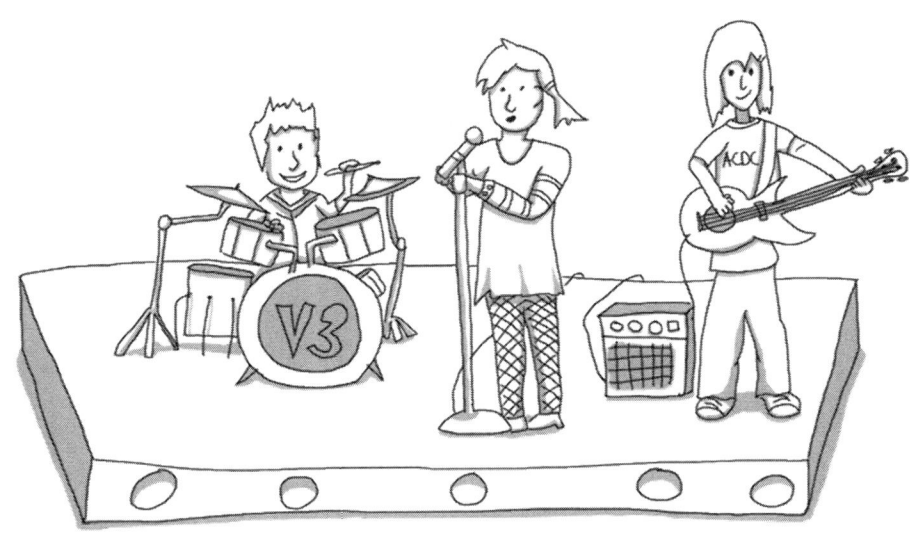

Have a band jam session

4. Have a pillow fight! Have a mud fight! Have a water balloon fight! Have a water gun fight! DO ALL OF THESE AT THE SAME TIME!

5. Play tourist in your own city.

   - Visit the tourist information center. Chat to the staff. Discover all the places you haven't discovered yet. Get a bunch of recommendations. Go explore! Get a paper map. Drive around or go on foot. Get lost. Get connected with the culture and history and ambience of the place you call home.

   - Plan a themed tour – peruse all the art galleries, or all the live music venues, or all the ice cream parlors. Hmm…ice cream…

   - Walk around an area you don't know. Try out a brand new restaurant, one you choose just by peeking through the window and digging the vibe.

   - Pretend to actually be from out of town and get people to give you suggestions of things to do or places to go. Adopt a fake accent. Develop an elaborate back story.

   - Challenge yourself to go into every single store in town. Just because.

   - Or simply go on a road trip through your own suburb and rediscover where you live.

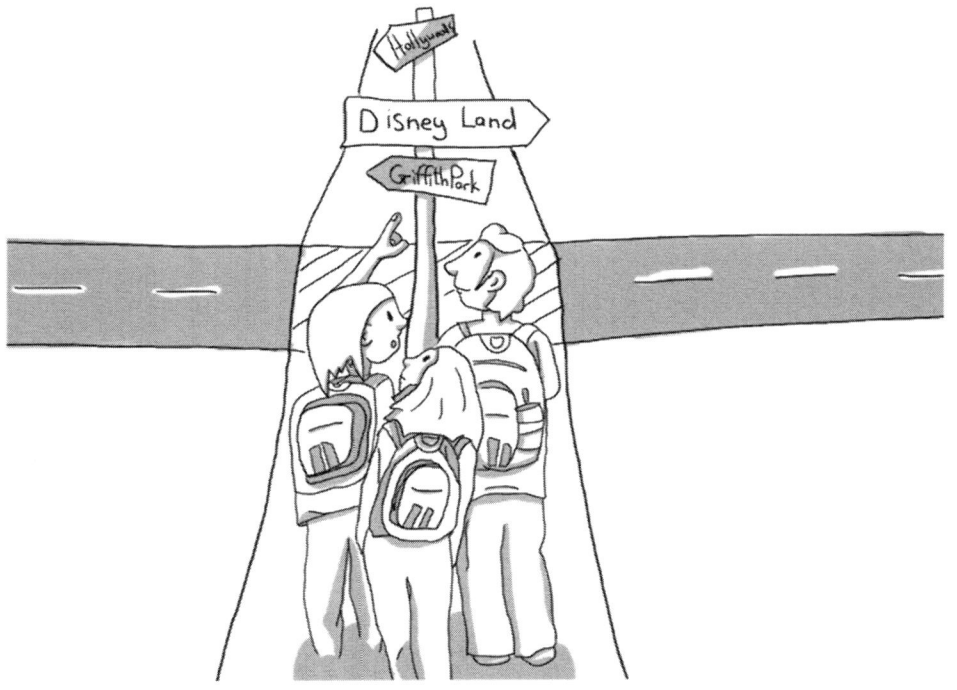

Play tourist in your city

6. Face time.

- Introduce yourself to your neighbor if you haven't already done so. Be awesome and bring over a gift too, like a batch of freshly baked homemade shortbread. If you're already acquainted, go over for a chat. Maintain the relationship. You don't have to make your neighbor a friend, but it's great to know there is someone right next door you can rely on in case of an emergency – and extend the same offer to them.

- Move into your best friend's house for a day (or more). If that's a bit extreme, then just hang out for a few hours, dude! Talk some nonsense, have a beer, take it easy.

- Surprise visit your best friend, or that grandma you haven't seen in an embarrassingly long time.

- Arrange a catch-up with an old college buddy.

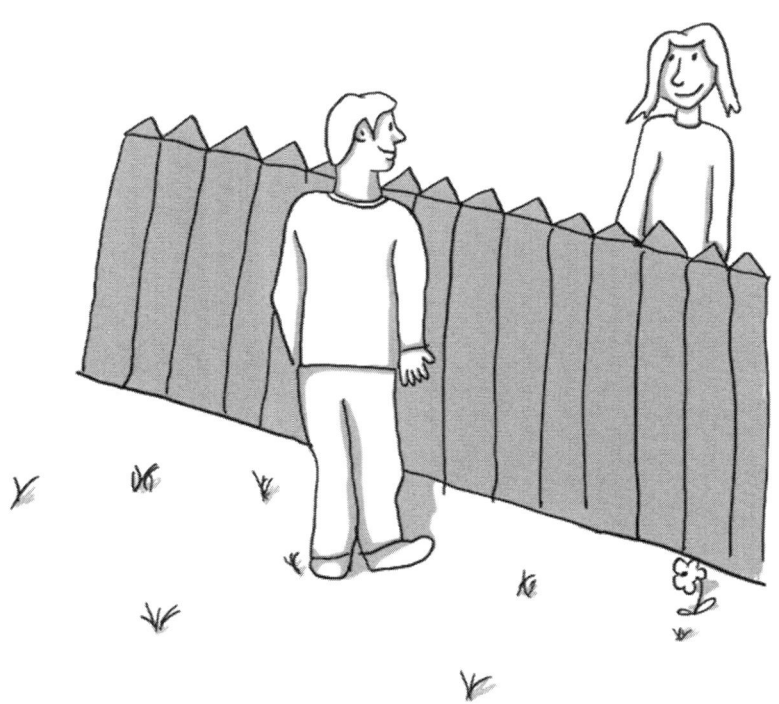

Chat to a neighbor

7. Share a moment with a stranger. Say hi to the haggard father sitting next to you on the bus. Wave at the old lady on the train. Smile at the angsty student. The moment when you make eye contact, the moment when their face softens - it's in that instant where the connection lives. Sure, it's just for a moment and you will both look away again. That's fine. Not every connection needs to be profound and lasting. Sometimes the small ones are just as powerful. Because that other person might be having a horrible day. And the moment you just shared with them lightened their load. And sure, you'll never know, but do this enough times and I promise you'll have made a difference.

8. Reply "attending" to your high school reunion.

9. Schedule a yacht cruise with all the cool kids, if you can swing it!

10. Volunteer yourself as the designated driver and chaperone your friends between several classy wine estates. Yes, you be the responsible one. Make sure they have a great time. Make their pleasure your priority.

11. Put a twist on the usual 'get together for drinks' meet-up: in honor of your smartphone detox, challenge your friends to all put their smartphones face down on the table. Now set this ultimatum - the first person who touches their phone has to buy a round of drinks for everyone!

12. Volunteer at an old age home, an animal sanctuary, a hospice, or a soup kitchen for the homeless. Be a good person. Be thankful for what you have.

13. Learn a few words in a new language. Continue to learn the rest of them. Find a language exchange partner. Take a trip to that country. Converse with the locals. Fall in love with the lifestyle. Uproot your life to emigrate. It could all start with a few words.

14. Make a family member's dream come true.

15. Adopt a pet from an animal sanctuary.

16. Support a community event - actually attend one of the local events advertised on that flyer you were given the other day.

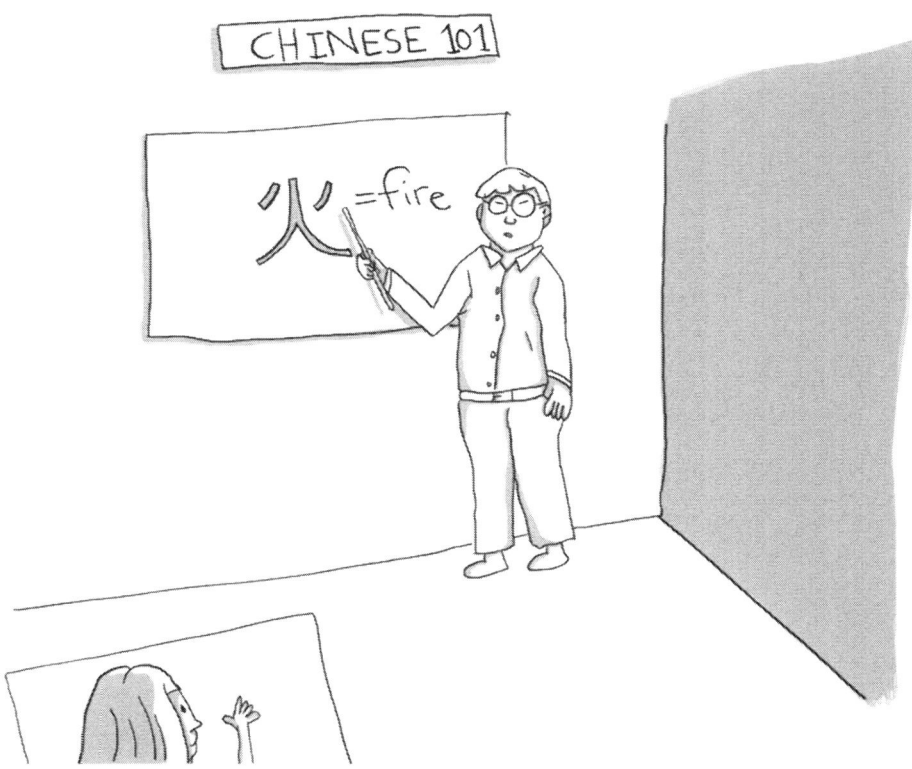

Learn a new language

Productivity

1. Re-organize your living space to serve specific functions - create a space in your home dedicated only to work/study. Create a totally separate space dedicated only to rest and relaxation.

2. Give your computer some love, service and attention.
   - Run a virus check.
   - Reorganize the mess of folders on your hard drive so that they actually make sense.
   - Defrag your hard drive.
   - Rename your photo albums logically.
   - Uninstall old, useless programs.
   - Unplug your desktop, take off the casing and dust the insides. Gross! Look at all that stuff!

3. Push yourself to exercise a little harder than you did yesterday. Do a few more reps, another round, pump your cardio for another thirty seconds. Start keeping track of every workout you complete, record what you did and try to push a bit more in every single session – even if it's just one more push-up. Having the evidence of your progress on paper is a massive morale booster.

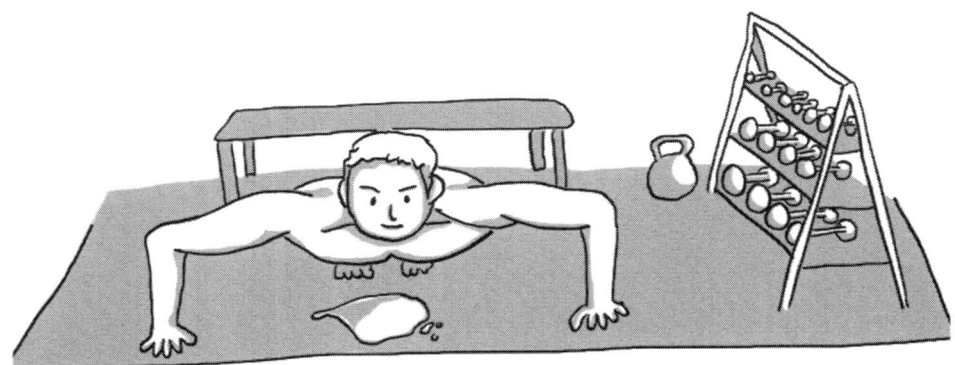

Workout harder today

4. Go for a jog *without* music. This time, let the environment be your soundtrack. Let in the bustle of the city streets, or the rustle of the forest. Enjoy the beat of your heart and the pounding of your feet on the pavement.

5. Purchase a legit swimming pool. Or settle for one of those little inflatable splash pools. Your last resort – the bathtub. Either way, find a way to dive into some water!

6. Sit down with an encyclopedia and don't get up until you have learned five interesting facts. Now find someone to enthrall with your newfound knowledge.

7. Teach an old dog new tricks. This may apply to your actual dog, but it may also apply to you.
   - Get super practical. Learn how to use those appliances you haven't got the hang of yet...how *do* you actually use all the settings on the washing machine? Read the manuals.
   - Sign up for a cooking class. Make your own pesto, bake your own bread, squeeze your own fresh orange juice. Learn to juice your own juice, and milk your own milkshake.

- Attend a seminar you know little about. Or attend a random, free one offered at the community hall. Purely for the novelty of it. Be open to the new information.

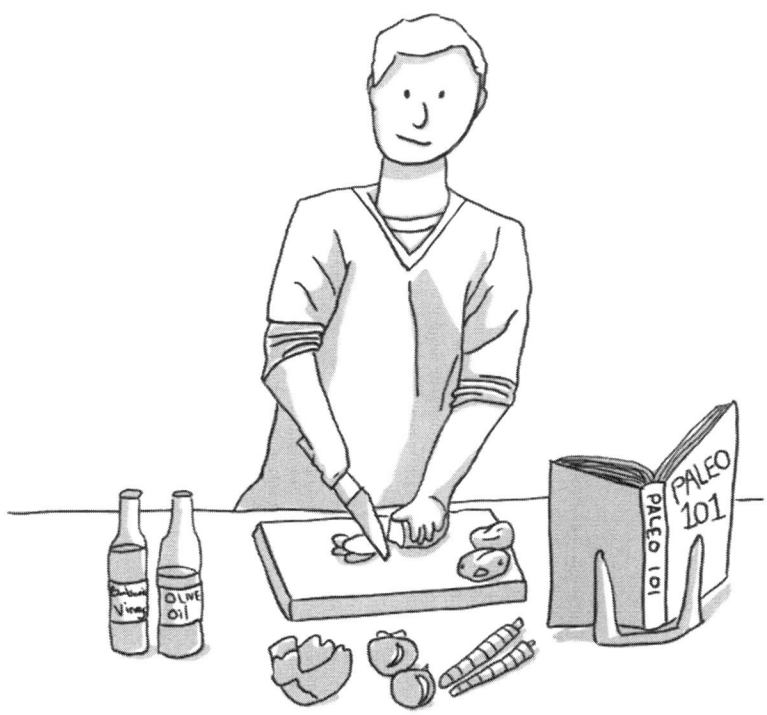

Learn to cook something new

8. Print and frame *real* photos. Of the family, or your trip to Vietnam, or your BFFs dancing in the rain that one time at band camp.

9. Plant something!
   - A tree.
   - A flower patch.
   - A bonsai cactus collection.
   - A herb garden.
   - A single square of lawn.
   - A vegetable garden.
   - If you already have one, go tend to it! Immediately! Weed it, water it, sing lullabies to the spinach!

10. Do some of the dirty work yourself.
    - Be your own garden service.
    - Clean all the monitors in the house.
    - Mow the lawn. Rake up leaves. Clean out the gutters. Chop wood. Water the cat. Fish the leaves from the pool.
    - Do renovations. Repair what needs a fix. Change the toilet seats. Visit a department store and gather some new ideas for your humble abode.
    - Build a shed and pave the garden.

- Repaint the walls *and* the fence. Clean the windows. Wash the dishes. Scrub the bathrooms. Spring clean. Do laundry. Change the sheets. Dust. Check between the couch cushions. Also wash the car. Afterwards you may collapse in exhaustion and simultaneously be struck by the realization of how your mom felt *every single day* while raising you.

11. Create some items which are uniquely you, and practical too. See how I rhymed that like a boss?
    - Take up pottery classes so you can handcraft your own crockery!
    - Make your own Christmas decorations.
    - Make fashion from scraps! Snip up those old jeans into cut-offs. Use that fabric you have squirreled away to make a scarf, or a tablecloth, or drapes.
    - Transform your old clothes in costumes for Halloween, or the annoying annual costume party you always get dragged to.
    - Finally learn how to sew a loose button back on.
    - Make your own soap, you hippy!

12. If you haven't already, seriously, learn to swim.

13. Hone, refine and brush up on some of your old skills.

14. Study for an upcoming test or exam. Or just study for the sake of studying.

15. Budget. See where you can save a bit. See where you can indulge a bit. See where you are wasting your resources – be it money, or time, or social energy. See where you are being inefficient.

16. Schedule a session in a floatation tank. Use it to quiet your mind, or use it to think clearly and lucidly on a single topic in a perfectly tranquil environment free of all distraction.

17. Spend an entire afternoon sifting through all the bric-a-brac at a garage sale. Or gather together all the *stuff* you have accumulated over the years - the stuff at the back of the cupboard, the stuff covered with the dust of disuse – and prepare for your own garage sale. Or just give the items away, perhaps to charity, perhaps to acquaintances you know will actually put a certain item to good use.

Entertainment

1. Get all artsy.

   • Paint flowers on your pot plants. On the pots, that is!

   • Find an article of clothing brilliantly white in color. Doodle all over it with permanent marker. Make a mess of it, or create an artistic masterpiece. Inspire a new fashion movement. Or just have some fun.

   • Doodle. Sketch. Scrapbook. Collage.

   • Paint. Paint with your fingers, or with your toes. Use an unexpected body part. Paint your own body, or paint a friend's face. Paint on a bowl, or a teacup, or an actual stretch of canvas. Practice perspective, depth, layering or abstraction in a detailed still life – or a nude study. Paint a nude self-portrait, or just paint while in the nude. Paint a wall. A cupboard. An old white shoe. Your entire house. Paint an epic mural on a decrepit community wall – this would be really cool to do with some friends.

   • Make something out of bits of wood and string and glue. An effigy. A voodoo doll. Go wild.

- Beat out your frustrations. Hammer nails into an old plank for no good reason at all! Or build something out of planks and nails. Saw through timber! DIY vintage shelf! *Make a rowboat!!!*

- Change is good. Rearrange an entire room, or all the stuff on your walls or shelves. Redecorate that tired corner of the lounge.

- Turn the everyday, the ordinary, into art. Use your recycling as raw material. Let your imagination know no bounds.

- Papier-mâché pottery.

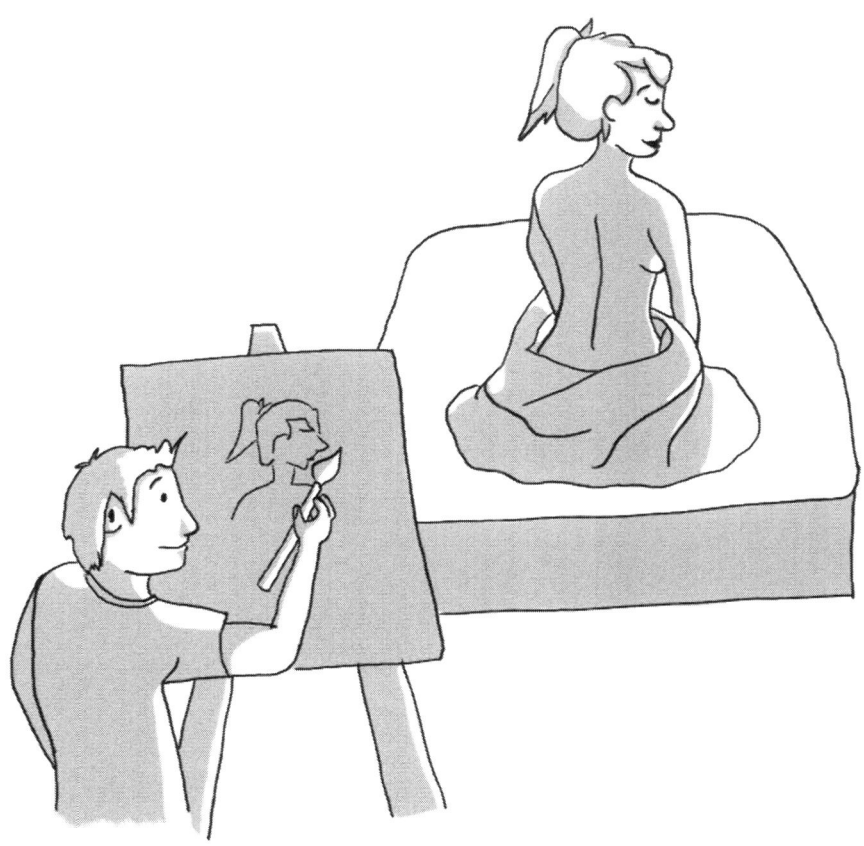

Hone a skill

2. Prank call a restaurant. Or prank the drive-through of a fast food chain. Walk through the drive-through but totally pretend you're driving.

3. Go skinny dipping. Solo, or with friends. Whatever. Have a great time. Don't get arrested.

4. Convert all your old CDs and video tapes to digital. Get with the times, dude. And have an amazingly nostalgic audio-visual journey through your past while you're at it.

5. Spend the afternoon/evening at a parade, or a fashion show, or the carnival. Ride a Ferris Wheel.

6. Enjoy the marvel that is nature: lounge at the beach, stroll through the botanical gardens, do yoga in a forest. Visit a natural hot spring. Go fishing. Sail on a rowboat. Simply walk barefoot on green grass, or drag your feet through warm beach sand.

7. Take up amateur bird watching. Try to identify the elusive little tykes by their unique calls.

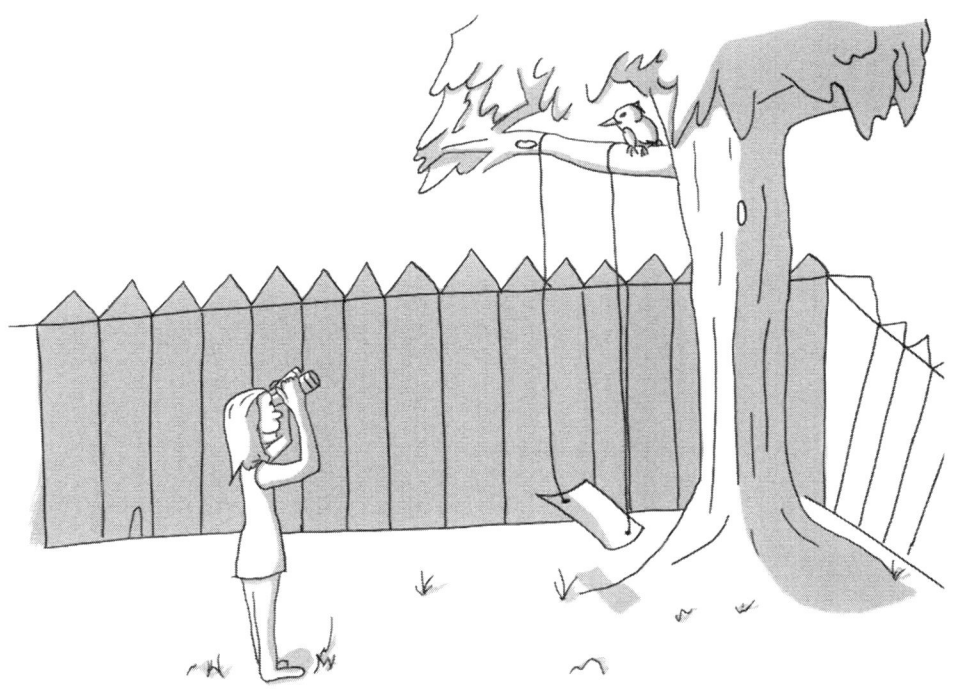

Take up amateur birdwatching

8. Visit a farm. Milk a cow by hand. Watch the chickens lay eggs. Charm the farmer and get treated to a donkey cart ride.

9. If you're loaded: fly in a hot air balloon. Or on a private jet. Drive in a limo. Go on a boat cruise, a helicopter ride, or on safari. Spend a night in a five star hotel.
   If you're not especially loaded: ride in a tuk-tuk, or on a horse. Spend a night in an affordable B 'n B.

10. Spend some hard-earned money on yourself. Decide on an amount, draw it cash, put it in an envelope titled "Me" and head out to the mall.
    - Go try on totally new clothes, buy a brand new outfit.
    - Replace a worn out pair of sneakers.
    - Buy a teddy bear.

    Alternatively, just window shop and spend nothing. Exercise your thriftiness. Resist temptation! Bring a friend with and fantasize about all the items you're *not* going to buy. Try on clothing, makeup and jewelry just for fun.

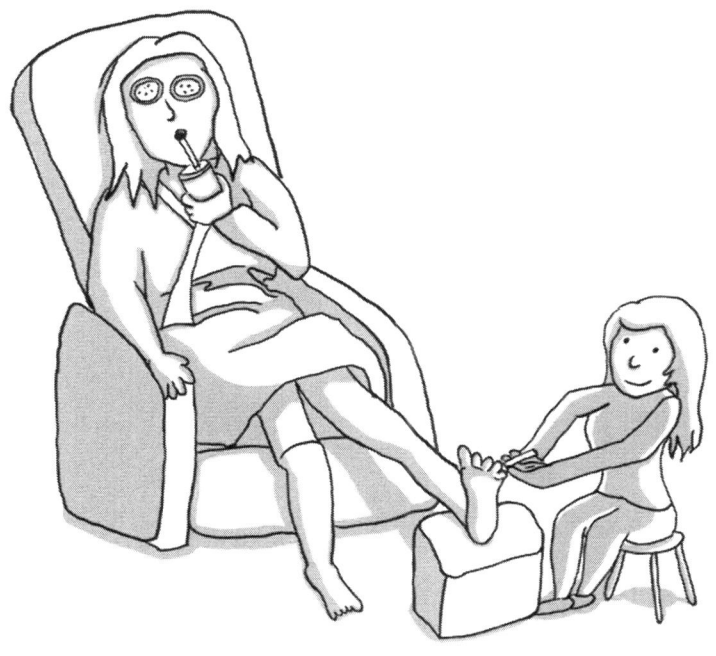

Spend $$ on yourself

11. Support a buddy at his sports match. Cheer until your lungs are on fire. Have a beer afterwards. Convince him he played like a legend even if he didn't.

12. Indulge your affinity for animals. Go to the museum, zoo, aquarium, or just to the pet store. Go whale-watching. See turtles hatch and run to the ocean.

13. Visit a graveyard.

14. Go to a Home Renovation Expo. Why not?

15. Blast music over the stereo. Dig out some old LPs. Dust off that old tape deck and go through your catalog of mixed tapes. Enjoy the bygones. Wallow in nostalgia. Try playing one of those LPs backwards to see if there are any hidden messages...

16. Go to the cinema and do a double movie marathon. Eat popcorn and drink a soda each time too.

17. Go to a nudist beach.

18. Level up your well-being. Suntan! Float in a pool! Eat good food! Sleep for a long time! Sleep in public!

19. Make yourself feel fabulous. Get a full body wax. A manicure. A pedicure. A facial. A spray tan. A day at the spa. Massages. Why not try a mud bath?

20. Waterworld!
    - Go for a swim in the ocean, at the community pool, or even just do some laps in your own pool you lucky fish.
    - Swim naked (at home!) or swim with your clothes on.
    - Pretend you're a dolphin.
    - Play Marco Polo, or force your friends to walk the plank.

21. Go outside. Into the garden. And then...
    - Climb a tree.
    - Build a tree house. Make it your special spot.
    - String up a hammock and spend lazy afternoons enjoying the sunshine.
    - Dig a deep hole. Just 'cause.

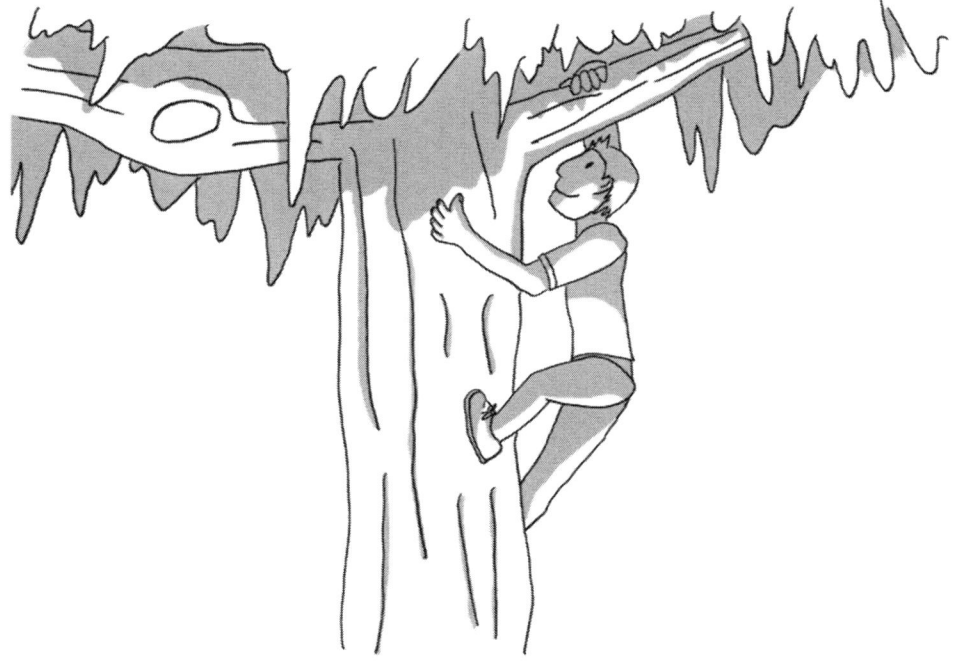

Climb a tree

22. Or get yourself to the park so you can:

- Fly a kite (that you've made yourself)!
- Play on the monkey bars, slide down the slide, swing on the swings. And, of course, seesaw on the seesaw.
- Fly your remote control chopper or terrorize folks walking their dogs with your remote control car.

23. Construct an indoor lab and conduct experiments like a mad scientist.

24. Play dress up. Or dress up your pet. Bonus points if you can get a tutu on your goldfish.

25. By now you're board (ahem).

- So start skateboarding, snowboarding or sandboarding.
- While you're at it you can build a snowman or a sandman.
- Just don't go overboard.
- If you get bored, why not play a board game in the snow, or on the sand? Tic-tac-toe would work perfectly...

26. Target practice!

- Line up empty cans and take them out with your slingshot, pellet gun or air rifle.
- Go to the shooting range. Fire real weapons.

- Become a legend at throwing stones with unnerving accuracy.
- Or just go practice darts in the garage.

27. Charge through the city exhibiting your sudden gift for parkour/freerunning/tricking.

28. Become a groupie for a band.

29. Hone your air guitar skills. Condition your headbanging muscle group.

30. Get off at a random bus stop or train station. Explore.

31. Dance in the rain. Definitely do this one without your smartphone.

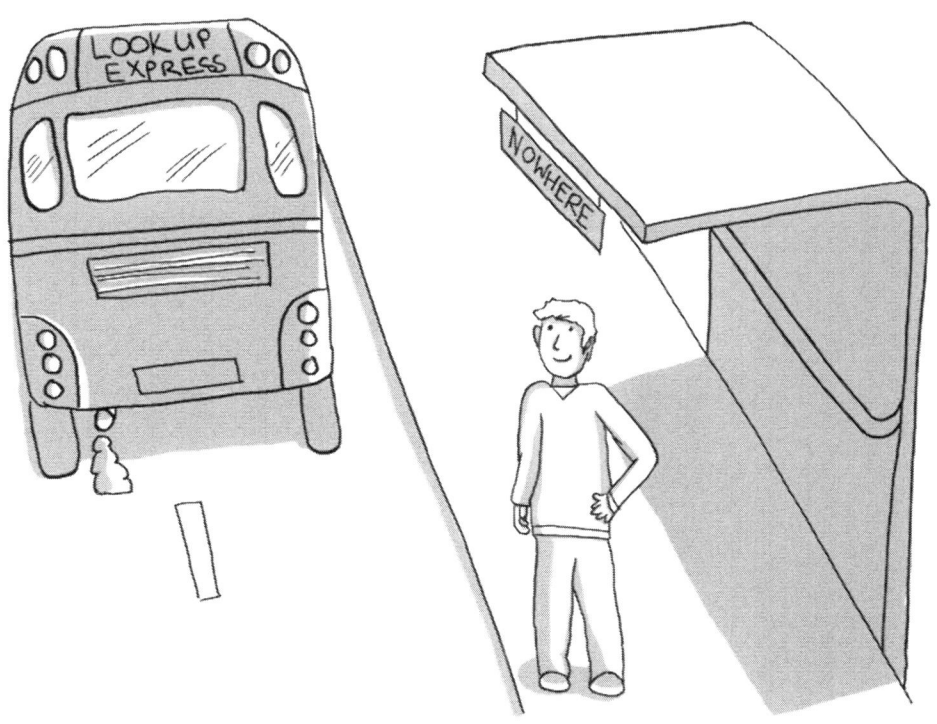

Get off at a random stop

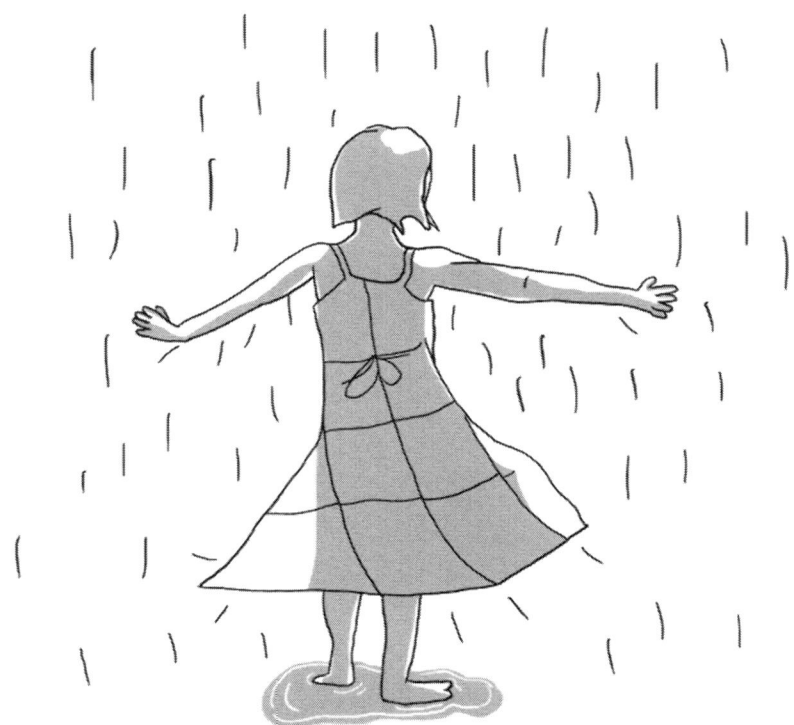

Dance in the rain

32. Make a drink of many flavors using everything you have in the fridge...

33. Crash some kind of party. Preferably a wedding.

34. Use red string to make an elaborate 'Laser Trap' all around your house. Try to navigate through the beams unscathed!

35. Dress up like a chicken. Strut around a fast food restaurant and yell: "You're eating my babies!"

36. Take photos in a photo-booth.

37. Jump in puddles.

38. Make sand castles or try to shape Nicky Minaj's rear end on the beach. Use the wet sand to make drip castles.

39. Make:
    - A miniature room out of a shoebox.
    - A ball out of elastic bands.
    - A sundial.
    - Balloon animals.
    - Carve a pumpkin.

- A scarecrow.

- A necklace out of cereal.

- A mosaic.

- A collage.

40. Of course, there are all the usual suspects...

- Cards (Rummy, Poker, Solitaire, ... ad infinitum)

- Board games (Cluedo, Monopoly, D&D, ... ad infinitum)

- Tug of War!

- Toss rings onto pegs, or horseshoes if you have them!

- Play bowls, or beach bowls.

- Slacklining.

- Juggling.

- Tap dancing.

- Walk on stilts.

- Yoga.

- Martial arts. Teach an effeminate buddy how to punch like Bruce Lee, grapple like a sumo and wheel kick like a ninja.

- Become a pro pogo stick jumper.

- Play hand tennis with a balloon, or bounce it between your friends without letting it touch the ground (try using *only* your head/nose/forearms).

- Learn to breathe fire. Responsibly.

- Play paintball, laser tag, air hockey, ten pin bowling, or miniature golf.

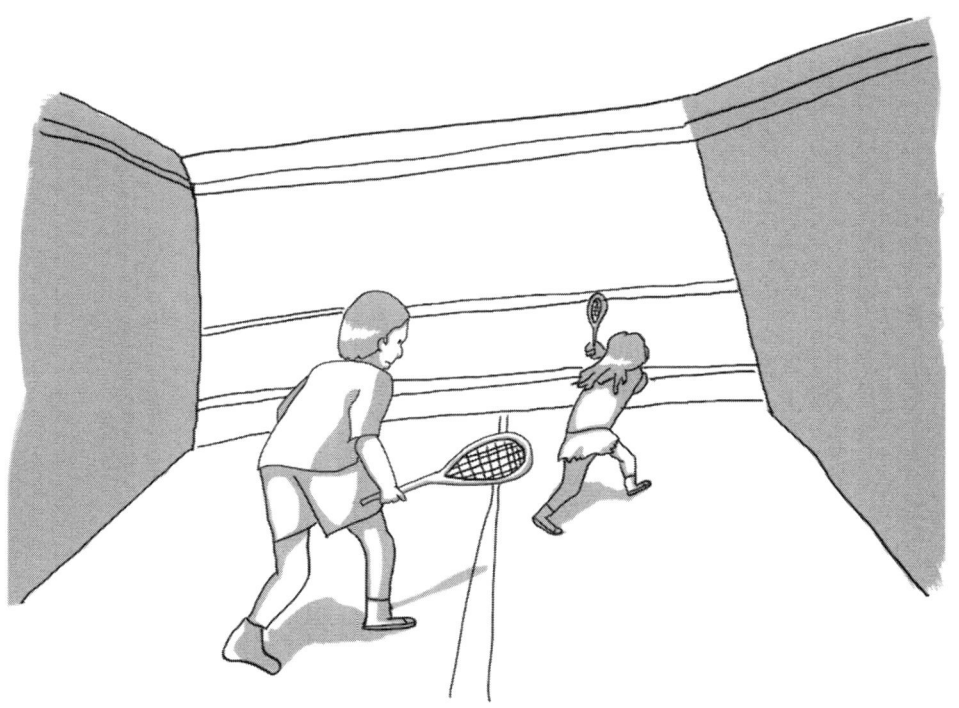

Play squash

Chapter 6 – Now that the stars are out...

You've nearly survived your 24 hour Thumbs Up challenge.

But the night is young and there's still so much more you can do!

Now is the time to begin winding down - or not! You can totally keep your energy going!

Your choice. Either way, you're nearly there!

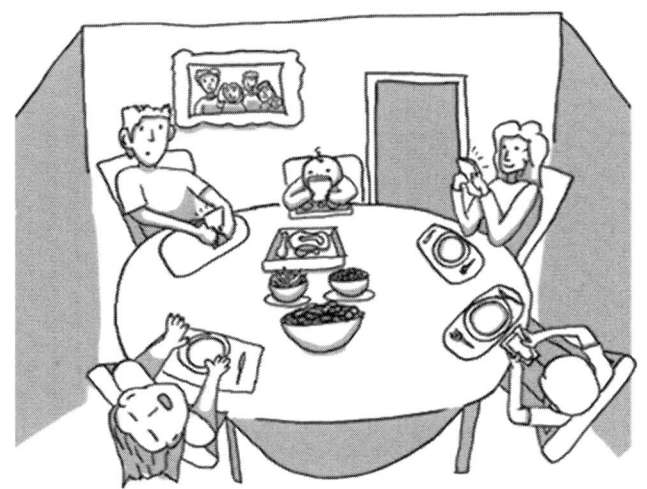

Before

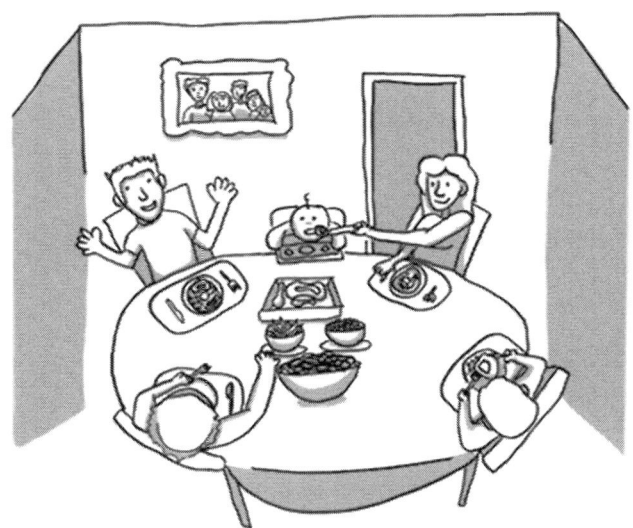

After

Connection

1. Enjoy the comforts of home, friends and family.

   - Invite way too many people over for a potluck dinner. Wear a white bib and don't stop eating until the bib is covered in food stains.
   - Hold a "Come Dine With Me" competition.
   - Partake in a "whodunit."
   - Host a themed movie night. Preferably with a massive projector screen and bottomless popcorn.
   - Get the whole family singing together.
   - Learn about your family history – a great opportunity to spend some time with grandma and grandpa.
   - Have a bonding session.

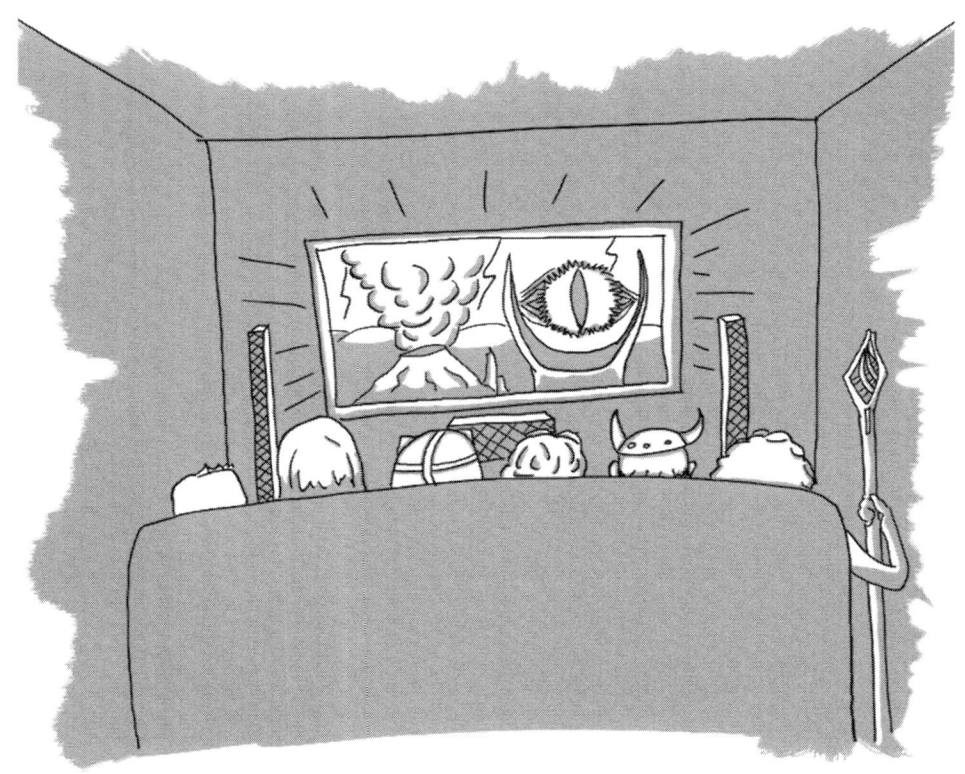

Host a themed movie marathon

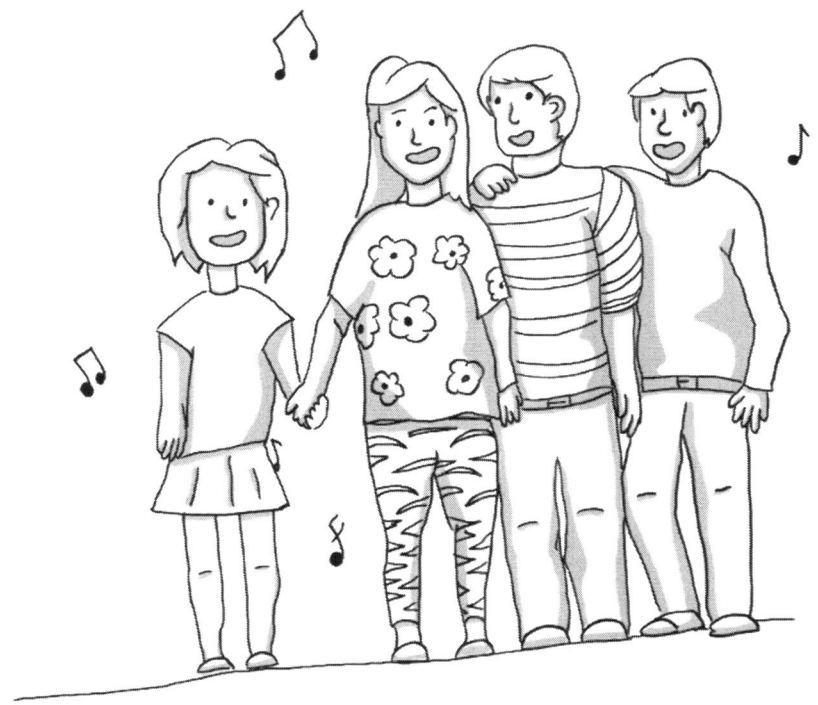

Get the family singing

2. Host a girls' night in. Go for a guys' night out where you try to get into the girls' night in.

    - Play Twister.

    - Play Truth or Dare.

    - The infamous 'closet kissing' game. A guy and a girl must go into a closet in the dark for a minute.

    - Play "Spin the Bottle" and indulge your teenage self.

    - Get a girl/guy's phone number the old-fashioned way – scribble it down on a napkin or in your classy moleskin notebook.

3. Start a book club.

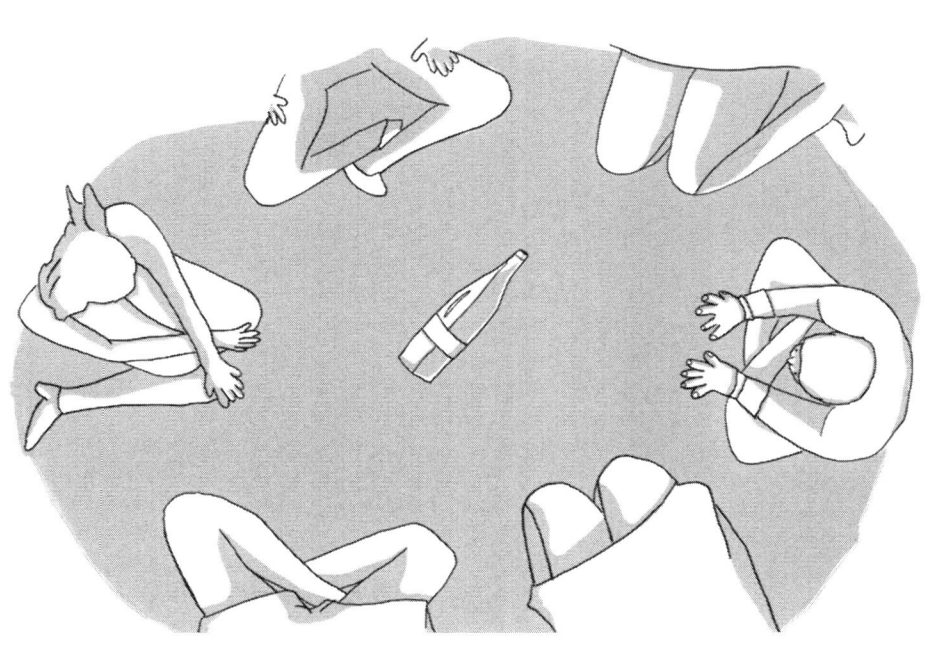

Play spin-the-bottle

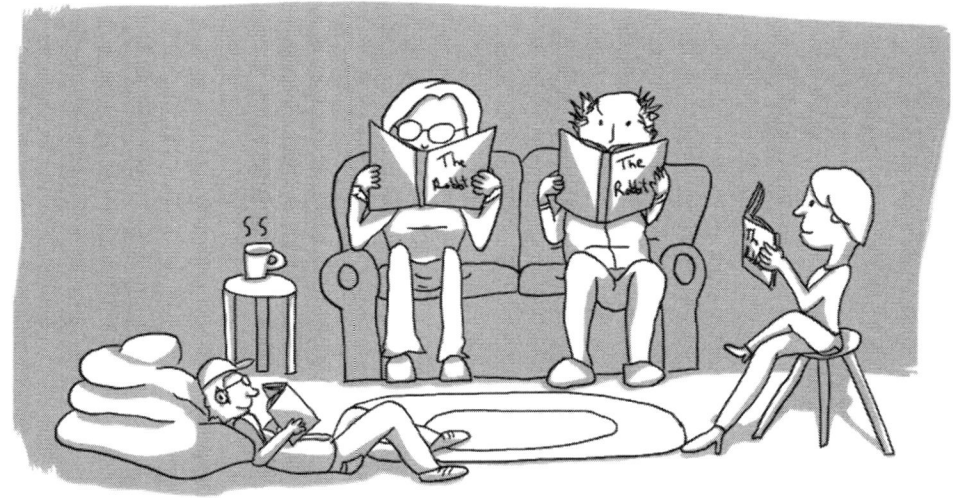

Start a book club

4. Play board games with friends. Get crazy. Buy a tabletop fantasy game like D&D. Dress up. Yell and whack each other with plastic swords.
    Invent a board game with insanely complicated rules.
    Better yet, make it a drinking game.

5. Gather together your bravest friends and spend a night in a haunted place. Play with an Ouija board. In the dark. At midnight. Wear disposable underwear.

6. Take someone up on that offer they made a while ago.

7. Arrange to see an old friend from college or high school.

8. Call up your bestie on the landline because it's cheap and just chat for an hour like you used to before there were smartphones.

9. Go on a blind date.

10. Have a candlelit picnic. If the weather is miserable, do it inside.

11. Figure out a way to scare your fearless friend or family member.

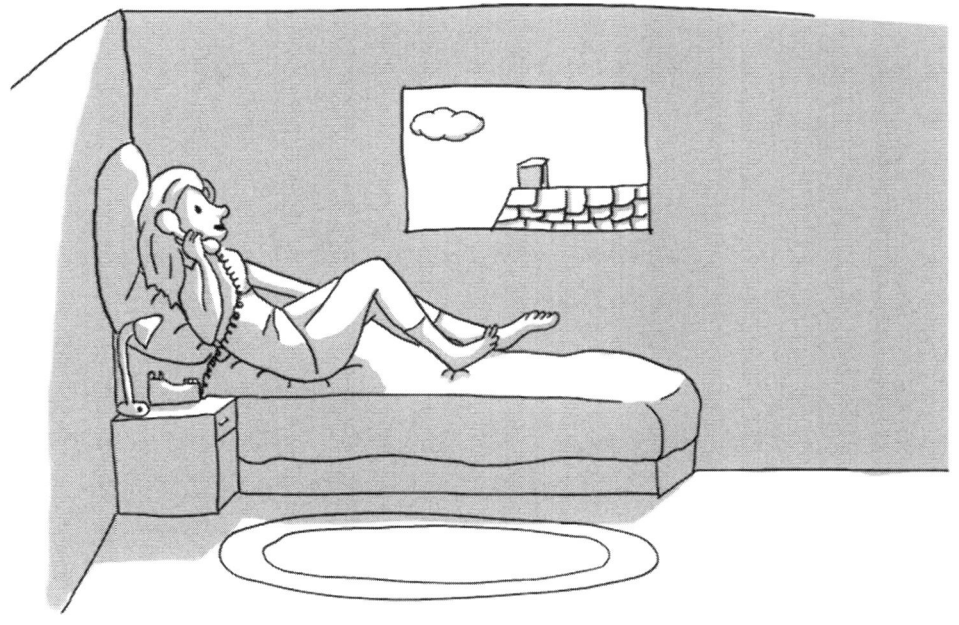

Call bestie on landline

Productivity

1. Go to a food fair instead of cooking dinner...or cook a gigantic meal and divide it up into portions for the entire week. Also, become a chopping master.

2. Burn all your old posters. This is both cathartic and industrious. While you're at it you may as well say goodbye to your old teddy bears.

3. Attend a speed dating event *in real life*.

4. Write out an entire notebook full of your favorite sayings.

5. Optimize your night life.
   - Remove all the technology from your bedroom
   - Set up blackout curtains.
   - Commit to a regular, sufficient sleep schedule.

6. Add a new dance move to your repertoire.

7. Begin a calming meditation.

8. Create a Zen garden.

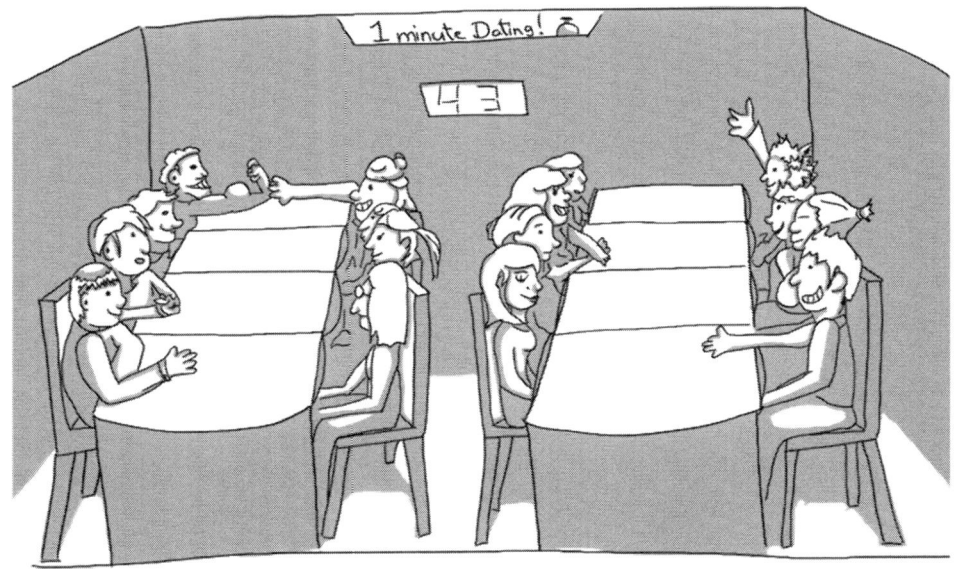

Attend a speed dating event

Entertainment

1. Watch the sunset.

   - As it dips towards the horizon build a bonfire and roast marshmallows.

   - Why not camp out right here in your own yard? Use it as a budget getaway for yourself or combine it with a romantic picnic…or you could totally just camp out in your living room and roast marshmallows in the fireplace.

2. Watch some theater. Dress up and pretend you're all fancy. Quote Shakespeare as much as possible.

3. Rock out at a concert. Headbang inappropriately during a live symphony orchestra.

4. Set off some fireworks purely for the fun of it.

5. Walk around the house totally naked. If you don't already do this on occasion, *now* is the time to enjoy this unexpected freedom.

6. Spend an evening stargazing. Get hold of a telescope if you can. You could make an entire event of it – snacks, blankets, a thermos of hot chocolate... Plan to see an eclipse or a meteor shower. Wish upon a star. Or just be amazed by a session at the Planetarium.

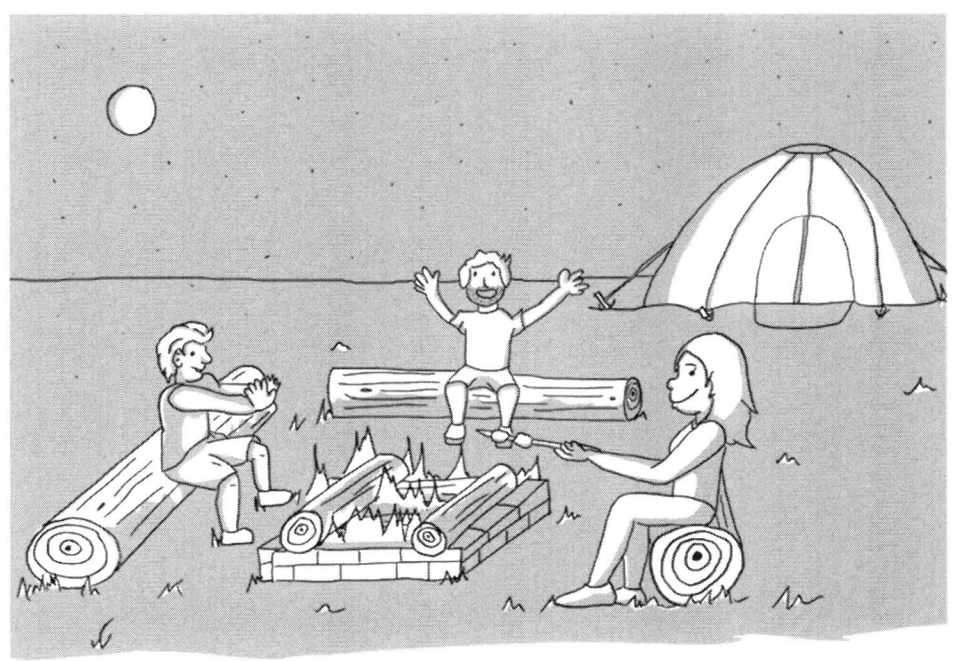

Roast marshmellows over a bonfire

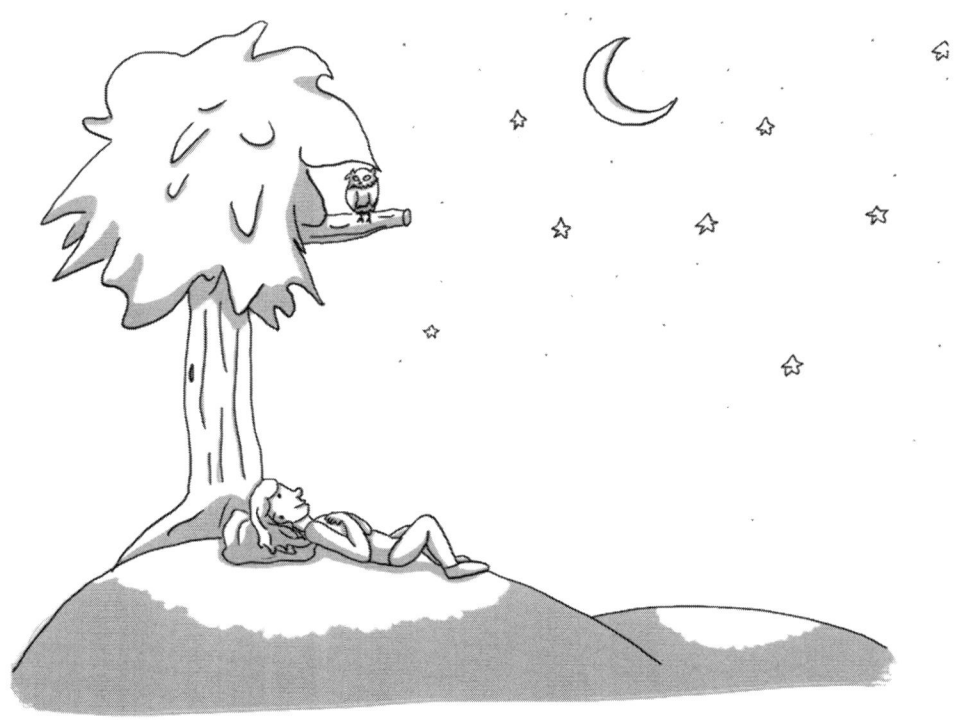

Lie down and gaze at the stars

7. Watch

    - a foreign film.

    - a banned movie.

    - some live stand-up comedy! YES!

    - a new TV series.

    - A mind opening documentary.

8. Read comics or magazines.

9. Drink a ridiculously overpriced bottle of champagne with a special group of peeps. Or just enjoy a cold beer. In the Jacuzzi.

10. Suit up in the perfect black suit.

11. Get hypnotized by a professional or dare one of your friends to have a go.

12. Create a family secret recipe! *Perhaps an entire book of these!*

13. Check what's in your neighbor's trash.

14. Free a lobster.

15. Tempt yourself to something (hmm...like triple choc fudge brownies) and then practice refusing it. Get *really* good at this. Then totally give in to the temptation and indulge yourself. Savor the flavor.

16. Create an obstacle course for your pets.

17. Just you and someone special. Share an umbrella as you stroll through the rain. Weather be damned. Share an umbrella as shelter from the summer sun. May no phone come between you!

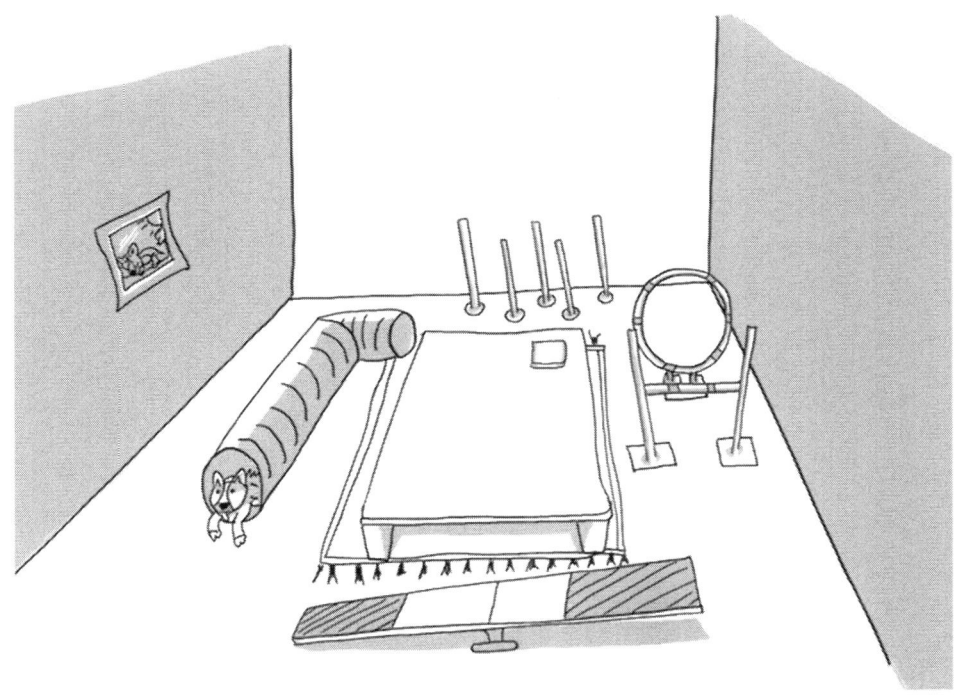

Create an obstacle course for your pet

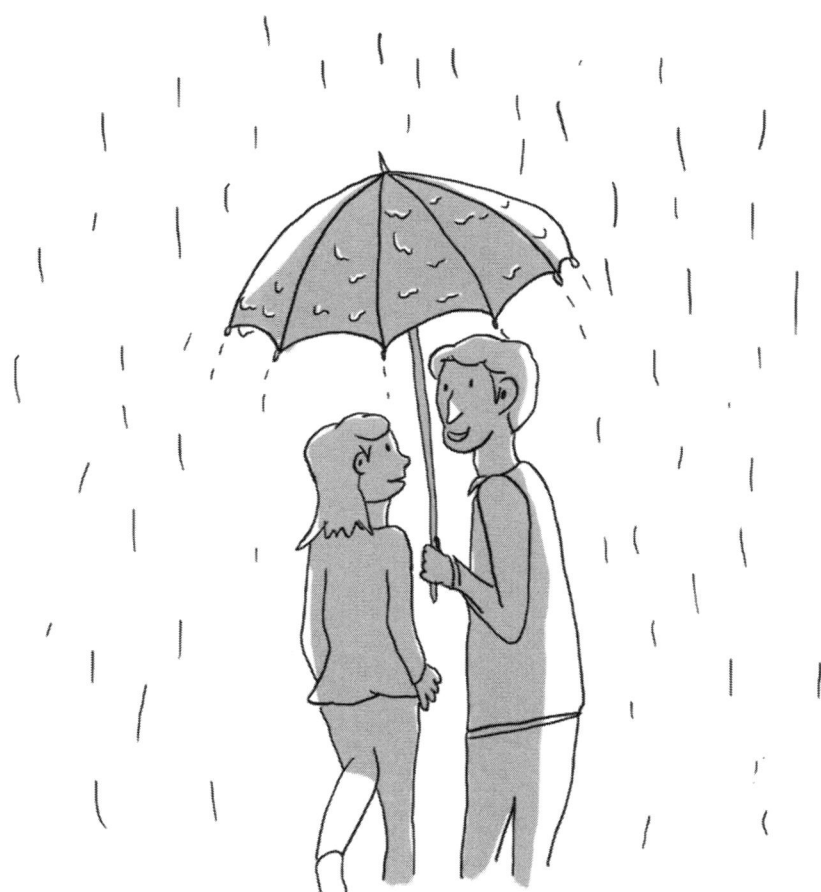

Share your umbrella with someone special

18. Get to the top of the highest building you can find and look down. Face that fear. And enjoy the view while you're up there, *without* taking photos. Enjoy it just for the sake of it.

19. Get a tattoo, even if it's just a temporary one.

20. Have a foam party.

21. Relive your childhood.
    - Build a fort with blankets and chairs to awaken your inner child. Make a den, your own secret hideout.
    - Continue to explore a childhood fascination – those comics you used to draw, or set up that old model train set again.
    - Flip through photo albums of you as a baby.
    - Re-watch video footage of your awkward early days.
    - Write your name on all your underwear with a permanent marker.
    - Go visit your childhood home. Drive through the streets you grew up in. Try to notice all the things that have changed. Notice how much *you* have changed.
    - Re-read your old favorites. You might be astounded at how differently you experience them now. Reflect on this.

22. Spoil that special someone. How about a romantic rooftop dinner? Or something as simple as a steaming mug of cocoa in front of a roaring fireplace. Perhaps a spontaneous picnic in the living room, or up on the roof.

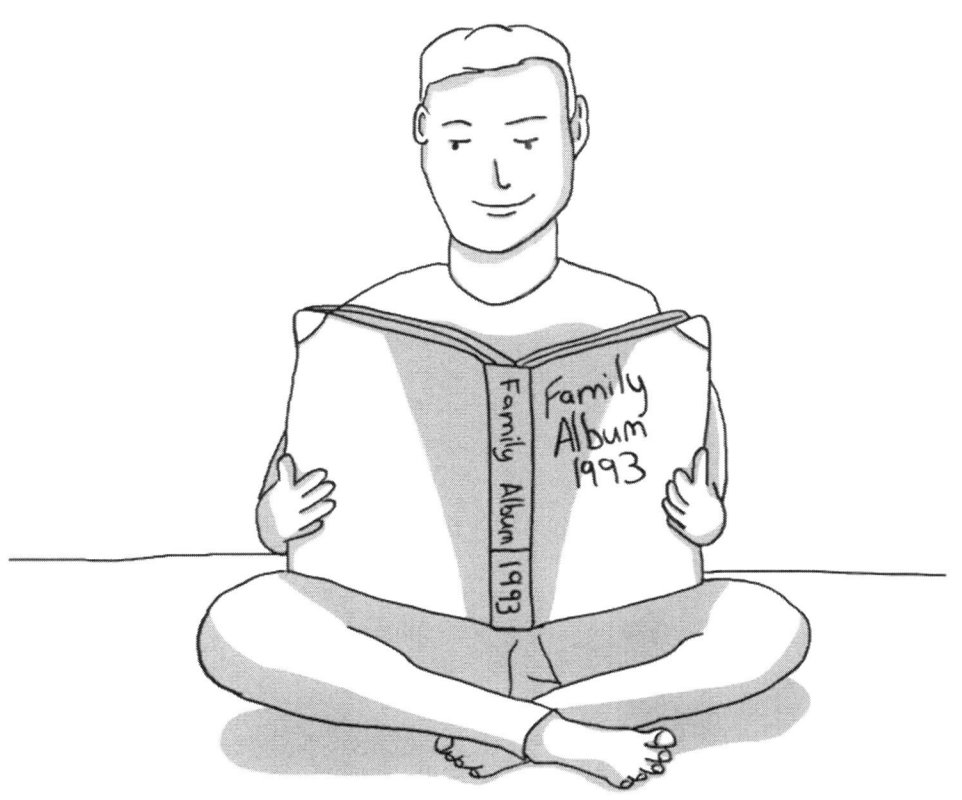

Check out old photo albums

Chapter 7 – Sleep tight.

This is it!

Choose a final activity before you slip into bed and enjoy your hard earned rest.

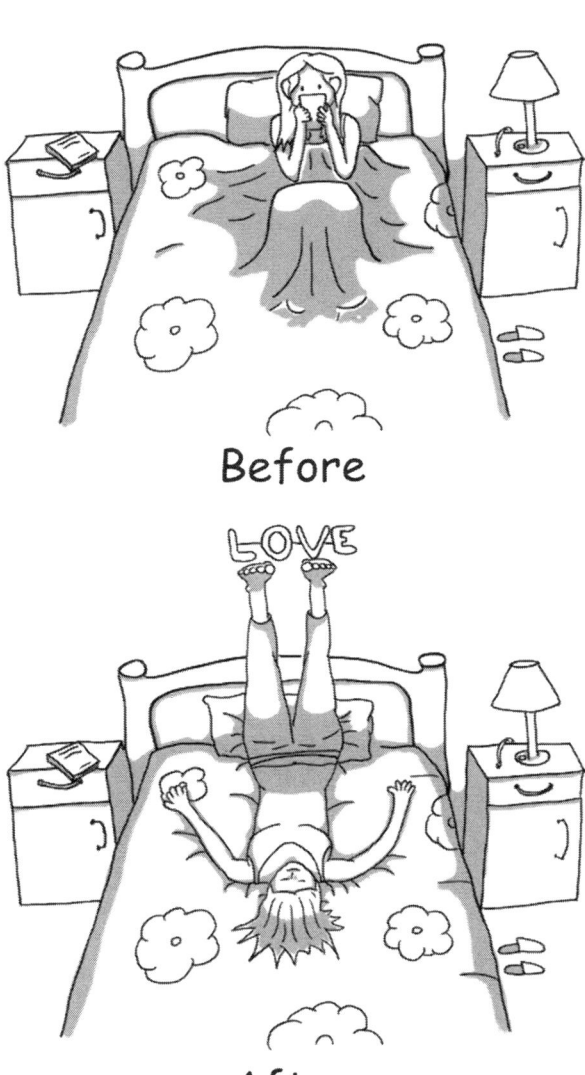

Before

After

Connection

1. Have a massage night with your partner. A foot and hand massage is super relaxing after a hectic day.

2. Tell your kids a bedtime story or phone a family member and get them to tell you a story.

3. Do a one minute meditation. Let go of all incoming thoughts. Make this a habit before you go to bed, try to go for one minute longer every night.

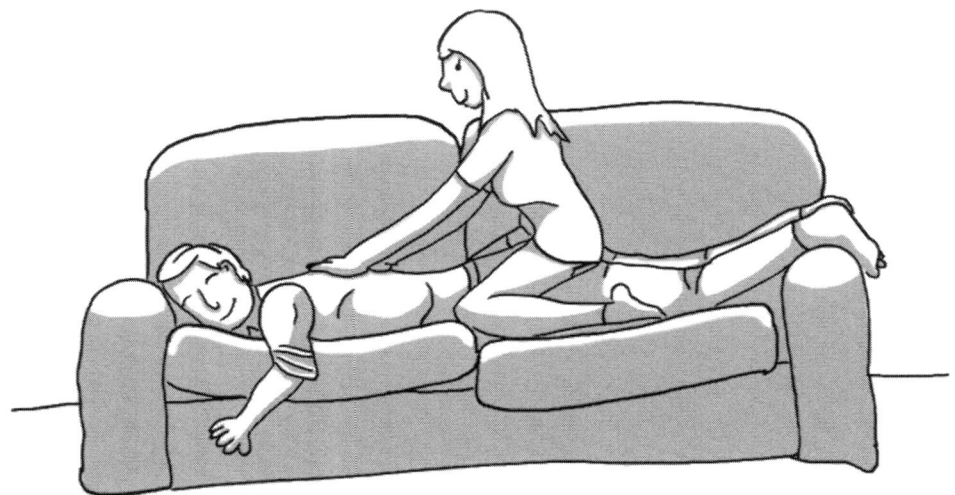

Have a massage night with your partner

Productivity

1. Pump up the positivity!

   - Write motivational messages to yourself and stick them up all over the house. Grab a marker pen and list your greatest strengths on the bedroom mirror so you see it first thing in the morning – and every time you look at yourself.

   - Write a letter to your future self detailing all the goals you are going to accomplish and all the adventures you are going to have along the way.

   - Read a success story, choose a role model and skim through their autobiography, picking out how you can apply their success to your own life.

2. Start a journal – why not begin by reflecting on your smartphone detox?

   - List the benefits and annoyances.

   - Explore the ways it made you appreciate the things you took for granted.

   - Detail what you liked doing the most, and what you're going to make more time for starting tomorrow.

3. Begin searching your soul.

4. Do a series of relaxing stretches.

5. List five things you're grateful for.

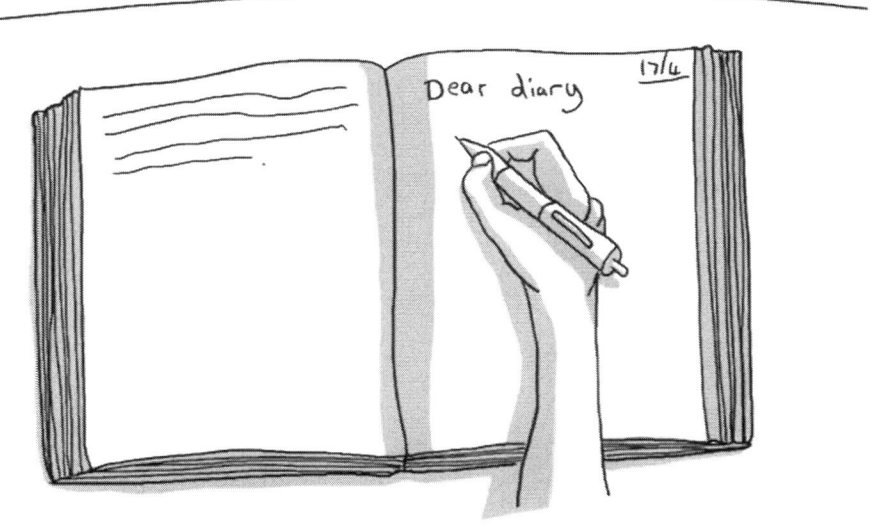

Start a journal

Entertainment

1. Flip through old photo albums. Or your school yearbooks.

2. Knit something.

3. Close your eyes and listen to soothing music.

4. Learn how to have a lucid dream. This takes work, but it is awesome once you can do it. Trust me!

5. Howl at the moon. Forget about your neighbors, purposefully shatter the sleepy silence, realize how awesome it feels to unleash the wolf inside.

6. Stay up all night. Because you can and nobody can tell you not to.

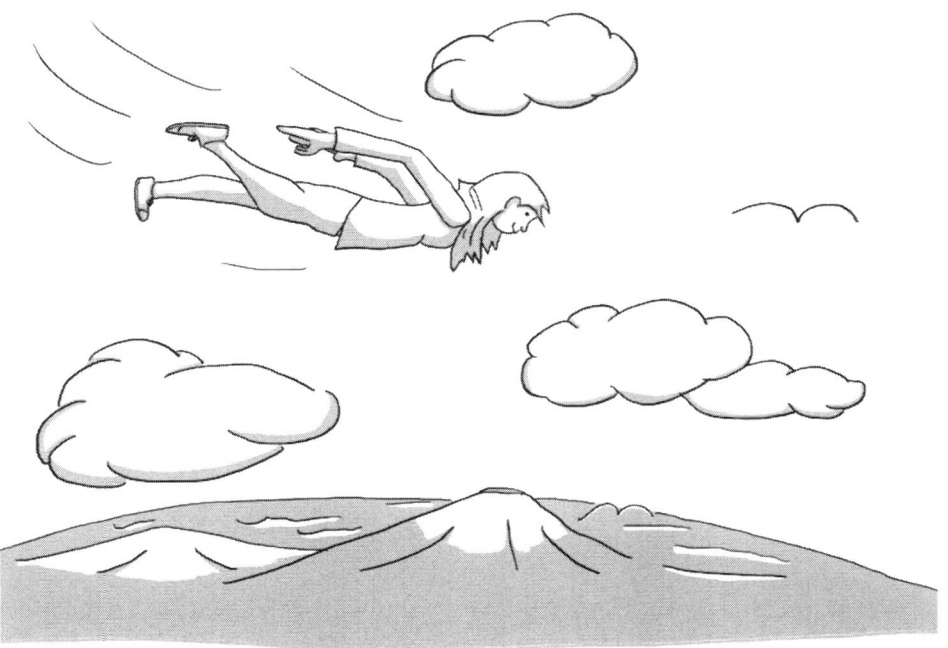

Try lucid dreaming

MISSION ACCOMPLISHED! Now What?

If you managed to survive without your phone for 24 hours then CONGRATULATIONS - you're one of the few who could.

You now have permission to turn your phone back on.

How long did you last? Now is the time to tell the world. Use this phrase:

"I survived the #24hourThumbsUp challenge for X hours!"

(If you haven't made it to the full 24 yet, don't sweat it! Now is your chance to try again! Keep going for just one hour longer.

There's a reason we called this a challenge!)

Once you've completed the full 24 hour challenge, have a breather. How do you feel? Spend the next few minutes reflecting on your experience.

Are you...

- energized and inspired?
- feeling like a new person?
- more aware of when to use your smartphone?

We sincerely hope you had a blast, and we'd love to hear how it went!

Email us at: 24hourThumbsUp@gmail.com

We're keen to share *your* stories as motivation for the Thumbs Up community! Pictures, words and videos – all these are welcome. Help us inspire the world! We want to share as many positive stories as possible.

- What did you get up to – which activities did you complete?
- What were the most difficult moments?

- Tell us about the top 3 benefits you experienced.
- Would you do the challenge again?

Awesome! The adventure is completed, but it's not the end of your Thumbs Up journey. We know it's impossible to stay unplugged. So plug *in* to the Thumbs Up community!

Check out our blog at: **www.24hourThumbsUp.com** (from there you can also find us on all the usual suspects including Facebook and Twitter).

We'll make sure you're up-to-date with new ideas for offline activities and share tips on a digital detox lifestyle. Here are some things you can immediately incorporate into your routine.

- Establish some 'coldspots' zones around the house. By this we mean areas where you don't allow smartphones AT ALL. Like at the dinner table.
- Take this a step further. Get a gadget which cloaks Wi-Fi signals to make it *impossible* to access the internet in a certain area.
- Hand in your phone before an event – ask a buddy to look after it so you can't be tempted.
- Set a curfew for checking emails.

- Put the entire family's phones in a shoebox after 8pm.

- Create 'lifestyle rules' for everyone in your house/office (no phones during mealtimes, etc.)

- Come up with 'taboos' amongst your friends and decide on all sorts of punishments for violating them. For example: while at a restaurant, get everyone to put their phone face down on the table. Whoever picks up their phone first has to buy a round of drinks.

- Buy less data for your phone or disable your data network when away from the office.

Lastly, THANK YOU for trying the 24 hour Thumbs Up challenge. Please continue to do the activities which inspired you!

SOS!

"Help! I'm having withdrawal symptoms! I need my phone to function as a human being!"

Don't panic. You're going to be just fine. Try these quick techniques to alleviate your agony:

- Breathe deep breaths, inhale through your nose, hold for 5 seconds, exhale through your mouth.
- Draw a picture of your phone.
- You need a substitute! Go buy a toy phone from a kids' store.
- Dunk your head in water.
- Grab someone and explain the pain you're going through.
- Write down your frustrations on paper. Pen an epic rant.

- Scream and shout!

- Last resort – assume the fetal position until help arrives.

Okay, seriously though…

Toughen up! You're nearly there. Look how far you've already come. Just stick with it. Jump right back into the chapter you're currently busy with and choose another activity to keep you going!

Bonus Chapter: Things to do with your phone when it's switched off...

1. Throw it at people to get their attention.

2. Use it as a paperweight.

3. Stare at your reflection in the blank screen.

4. Get ridiculously good at balancing your phone on the tips of two pens. Impress your friends, family and colleagues and then become a YouTube sensation.

5. *Pretend* to make a call. See how long you can get away with

this for.

6. Disassemble it and put it back together again. Take a look at the inner workings of this wonder of science and technology. While you're at it give the thing a thorough cleaning.

7. Make your own cover, or redecorate the one you already have. Carve, paint or draw a super cool design on it.

8. Use your phone as a ruler. Draw straight lines.

9. List all the complaints you have with this model. Then how about *you* try and come up with a new design which rectifies all these flaws.

10. Stash away a note inside it like a high-tech message in a bottle.

Another Bonus Chapter: How to get rid of your smartphone – permanently.

So you've enjoyed your Thumbs Up challenge. You've enjoyed it so much you've decided to never use a smartphone again. Good riddance to the little radiation cube!

Here are some inventive ways to annihilate it.

1. Use your phone as a target at the shooting range. The budget version of this is to just throw rocks at it.

2. Paint all over it and put it on your mantelpiece. Let this be a bold statement for your new anti-tech way of life! Grow your

hair go live on a commune. Plant your own parsnips.

3. Test how waterproof your phone is. Use it as a coaster. Boil it in the kettle. Drown it in the bath. Flush it down the loo like a *really* expensive goldfish.

4. Find ways to determine just how scratchproof the screen actually is.

5. Drop it from higher and higher places until it shatters into satisfyingly small pieces.

6. Disassemble your phone into its component parts and use these to create a postmodern masterpiece which sparks a revolution in the hearts and minds of an entire nation and eventually leads to world peace and the Age of Aquarius. Then fashion your masterpiece into a crude crown and rule the free world...Pinch yourself. Wake up. Realize you've just ruined your phone for good. Celebrate your achievement.

7. Use your phone to play 'catch' with your dog.

8. Glue your charger to your phone and swing it around, yelling like a medieval warlord. Then smash the damn thing against the wall!

9. Toss your smartphone into the blender and see which one breaks first.

10. Bake it into a cake. Surprise!

This is the end. For real. If you still want more, continue

the adventure at: **www.24hourThumbsUp.com**

18732669R00115

Printed in Great Britain
by Amazon